Self-Mutilation

Self-Mutilation

Robert Robertson Ross
Hugh Bryan McKay
University of Ottawa

Lexington Books
D. C. Heath and Company
Lexington, Massachusetts
Toronto

Library of Congress Cataloging in Publication Data

Ross, Robert Robertson.
Self-mutilation.

Bibliography: p.
Includes index.
1. Self-mutilation. 2. Adolescent psychiatry.
I. McKay, Hugh Bryan, joint author. II. Title.
RJ506.S44R67 616.8′582 77-18681
ISBN 0-669-02116-4

Printed simultaneously in Canada

Printed in the United States of America

International Standard Book Number: 0-669-02116-4

Library of Congress Catalog Card Number: 77-18681

Contents

List of Tables

Acknowledgments

Several years ago the Department of Psychology at the University of Waterloo began to collaborate with the Ministry of Correctional Services of the Province of Ontario in providing treatment and research services to an institution for behaviorally disordered adolescent delinquent girls: Grandview School. Through this collaboration a teaching hospital in corrections was developed in which faculty members and graduate students could work together with the staff of the institution in an attempt to develop innovative and efficacious strategies for the management and treatment of behaviorally disordered adolescents. The initial development of this cooperative enterprise was encouraged by Drs. R.H. Walters and H. Lefcourt of the University of Waterloo and L. Hackl, D. Sinclair, and the Honorable A. Grossman of the Ontario government.

The treatment-research project described in this book comprises one aspect of this long-term cooperative enterprise. The research and the preparation of the manuscript were supported by the Ontario Ministry of Correctional Services; the Ontario Mental Health Foundation (Grant # 200); and the Faculties of Graduate Studies and Social Sciences of the University of Ottawa.

Although we share the authorship of this volume, there are numerous individuals who shared our concern for its theme over the years, and their contributions were essential to the development of our treatment-research work and the subsequent preparation of this manuscript.

Drs. Ken Bowers and Don Meichenbaum, who served as consultants to Grandview throughout the project, provided invaluable advice, encouragement, and stimulation.

We are most grateful to the Research Division of the Ministry, and particularly to A. Birkenmayer, for continuing support, assistance, and encouragement of our research.

A large number of people assisted in our research over the years: S. Bartlett, A. Bratasiuk, C. Binnington, N. Bowen, S. Breault, K. Doody, L. Futcher, M. Gauley, C. Humphrey, N. McConkey, M. Taub, P. Trantina, and R. Wreford.

We are particularly grateful to W.R.T. Palmer and C. Kenney for their extensive assistance in the preparation of the research reported in chapter 6 of this volume. Portions of this research have been published in the *Canadian Journal of Criminology*, 1978, 20: 375-392, and we would like to thank the editor (Mrs. Hilda Davy) for her kind permission to reprint parts of it here. We also appreciate the permission of the editors to reproduce in chapter 7 of this volume portions of the research which has been published in *Canada's Mental Health*, 1976, 24(2): 15-16. A special note of gratitude is extended to B. Krug-McKay for her invaluable assistance in preparing chapter 5 and her many helpful suggestions on earlier versions of this manuscript.

We gratefully acknowledge the assistance throughout the years of the many members of the psychology department at Grandview who contributed to our treatment programs: B. Augustine, B. Bradley, R. Cannon, T. Hayachi, G. Johnston, W. Palmer, M. Pruesse, E. Staples, and J. Sherman.

We are grateful for the secretarial assistance of R. Bertrand, E. Champagne, C. Hoang, W. MacDonald, and A. Taylor.

We express our sincere appreciation to the superintendent of Grandview and his medical, psychiatric, social work, teaching, and correctional staff and to the host of volunteers, student nurses, and interns who assisted in our treatment-research project.

We omit many whom we have attempted to thank individually over the period of this work and take this opportunity to thank them once again, collectively.

Finally, we wish to thank Tom Loker, Walter Wright, Bob Smith, and the girls at Grandview from whom we learned so much.

Prologue: "To Mom with all my Hate."

Debbie was fifteen when she first arrived at the training school. Isolated from her parents, her sisters, and her baby brother; chastised by a well-meaning but "no other recourse" judge; discredited by her probation officer whom she thought was her friend; cut off from her friends—the "bad companions" whom mother blamed for Debbie's problems; and permanently separated from her boyfriend, Debbie was lonely, depressed, angry, bitter, and resentful. As her probation officer drove her from juvenile court to the training school, the tears Debbie shed were not designed to impress him or to make him feel guilty for having recommended training school. Debbie could produce crocodile tears at will, but there could be no doubt that this time Debbie's grief was genuine. She had been warned many times that her behavior would lead her to training school, but the warnings had had little impact on her adolescent mind. They may even have urged her on.

As the station wagon approached the training school, Debbie's tears dried and her sadness gave way to a much more adaptive emotion: fear. She had heard about training schools: junior jails, rigid discipline, uniforms, amazon matrons, cells, isolation, brutality, homosexuality.

In the reception center the staff tried to make her feel at home: "It's up to you how long you have to stay here," "We are all here to help you," "Just do what you are told and earn your credits," "It's all for your own good," "It's up to you," "Acting up just leads to more time," "We just want to help you," "Just keep your nose clean," "Just mind your manners and do what you are told," "There's no sense in fighting it," "Cooperate," "We understand." The same advice couched in more professional language she heard from the social workers, psychologists, and psychiatrists who welcomed her, then probed into her background and her personality for some pathology that would explain her behavior. "We are only trying to help" were the lines of the chorus, repeated in unison.

The professionals started on her in the reception center—the assessment unit. Interviews, conduct ratings, social histories, and educational tests were administered during a two-week onslaught which left her more perplexed than ever about who she was, why she was there, and what was going to happen to her. The reports could have told her if she had been allowed to see them.

---

[a]Author's note: In order to ensure the anonymity of this case we have used a fictitious name and altered several aspects of "Debbie L.'s" history.

Social History Report

Debbie L. is an attractive fifteen year old from Mississauga, a suburb of Toronto. At admittance she was wearing an excessive amount of make-up and her fingers were badly stained with nicotine.

Debbie is a 5-foot 5-inch blonde girl who has pleasant features and a ready smile. Her complexion is rather poor, and she will likely require some dental work for cavities. Since admittance she has shown considerable interest in her appearance and arrived for all interviews neatly dressed and well groomed.

Debbie is the second in a sibline of five; three younger brothers and one older sister. Her father, aged forty-two, is a truck driver. He is presently unemployed. Her mother, aged thirty-seven, is a hairdresser. She is presently unemployed and living on welfare. Debbie's parents separated some six years ago when Debbie was nine. There have been several attempts at reconciliation but each ended after major quarrels brought on by her father's excessive drinking. With the exception of a six-month period when she stayed with the maternal grandmother, Debbie has always lived with her mother. Debbie's oldest sister, age eighteen, is currently employed as a salesclerk in a department store and plans to marry in three months. Debbie's brothers, aged thirteen, eleven, and nine, live at home and attend school. None of her siblings have had contact with juvenile court. However, her oldest brother, Richard, has been suspended from school on two occasions for fighting.

The family home is a comfortably furnished semi-detached three-bedroom house which is badly in need of repairs. Debbie's mother complains that she is unable to maintain the house in reasonable condition on the limited income she obtains through welfare. The father provides some support for the children, but only sporadically. Mrs. L. feels she would rather spend her meager resources on good food and clothing for the children. The older sister contributes some money to the home for room and board. Her mother has been unable to work at all in the past eighteen months because of an arthritic condition which prevents her from standing for any length of time.

Mrs. L., though somewhat overweight, is a very attractive woman who speaks fondly of all her family and is obviously distraught about Debbie. She has visited Debbie three times since her admission to training school two weeks ago. However, she feels she will be unable to visit very often because of limited finances. (We have contacted the Family Service Bureau to determine whether they might provide an assessment of the home with a view to providing family therapy.)

Mrs. L. describes Debbie as a normal healthy girl who presented no problems in the home until she entered grade eight. Her early life was uneventful. She was reported to be progressing well at school during the early grades and was described by her teachers as an outgoing pleasant girl who made friends easily. They felt that she demonstrated leadership qualities. She was actively involved in school sports, enjoyed ballet and tap-dancing classes at the YMCA, and sang in the church choir with her sister. The school reports revealed no indication of behavior problems until grade eight. Her failure in grade seven can be attributed to the fact that her mother had moved frequently, and she was required to change schools. She was also absent from school on a number of occasions during that year. However, reports from her grade eight teachers made several references to disciplinary problems–inattention, foul language, and poor work habits. In addition, she was truant on several occasions. On one occasion she was absent from school for two weeks and gave her teacher a note to which she had signed her mother's name. Debbie's mother claims that this was the first time that Debbie had ever been dishonest, and she was at a loss to explain her behavior. However, she noted that Debbie had been "spending too much time" with some boys from the local high school whom Mrs. L. thought were much too old for her. Mrs. L. had reprimanded Debbie and forbidden her to see these boys. At the insistence of Mrs. L., the principal arranged to have Debbie referred to the school psychologist. She was seen on three occasions at guidance clinic in November.

The following summarizes the psychologist's report: "Debbie is a charming and articulate adolescent who is presently functioning at the superior range of intelligence (WISC) . . . Personality testing (TAT, Rorschach, HTP) yields no evidence of psychopathology. The personality profile is well within normal limits and consistent with that of a fourteen-year-old adolescent girl . . . She is experiencing some conflict with her mother's imposition of controls which Debbie perceives as overly restrictive and childlike . . . She appears to have failed to reconcile herself to her father's absence and is frustrated by what she perceives as his inability to express affection towards her . . . Debbie's present difficulties appear to be related to conflicts in the home, to her recent transfer to a new school with resulting academic problems, and her mother's attempts to isolate her from her friends. It would seem appropriate to have Debbie and her mother seen again in the near future with a view to reassessing their relationship. . . . Suspension from school is contraindicated in this instance and teachers should be encouraged to involve Debbie in all school activities."

In the interview with the psychologist Debbie claimed to have consumed alcohol on several occasions and to have experimented with marijuana. It was also reported that she had been involved with boys much older than herself but denied having had sexual intercourse. The psychologist concluded that Debbie's problems were consistent with a diagnosis of "Adjustment Reaction of Adolescence."

Debbie appeared to improve both at school and at home following her contact with the guidance clinic. However, two months later she was apprehended by the police following complaints from local merchants about the behavior of a group of teenagers in a neighborhood plaza. Debbie was taken home, and her mother grounded her for three weeks. Apparently in response to the grounding, Debbie was again truant on several occasions. She was suspended from school in April following a two-week period of truancy. Mrs. L. imposed greater controls on Debbie at this point, but three weeks later Debbie ran away from home.

She was apprehended soon after with a gang of youths who had been staying in a summer cottage at Barrie, Ontario. Apparently the cottage had been vandalized, and there was evidence of both alcohol and drugs. Debbie apparently had been sexually involved with at least three of the boys during the five-day stay at the cottage.

In May Debbie appeared in Metropolitan Toronto Juvenile and Family Court charged with unmanageability, including sexual immorality (Debbie claims she was charged with "sexual immortality"). Considerable concern was expressed by the court about the conflict between the reports of Debbie's behavior and the impression she created as a bright, socially alert, normal, and healthy teenager. Assessment at the Juvenile Court Clinic corroborated the findings of the earlier psychological examination and yielded no evidence of psychopathology. The court placed her on probation for one year and returned her home to the care of her mother. During the first few weeks of her probation Debbie made remarkable improvements in her relationship with her mother and appeared to be adjusting well. She related very well to her probation officer and reported regularly. However, in June Debbie began staying out overnight and refused to account for her whereabouts and was totally indifferent to her mother's reprimands. When returned to the court Debbie was flippant and unrepentant and refused to accept her mother's restrictions. The judge placed her in a foster home with Mr. and Mrs. S.G. Debbie's initial adjustment in this home was satisfactory, but she continually complained of being homesick. Thus she was allowed to visit her home on weekends, but the relationship was so strained that on one occasion her mother refused to allow her into the house. That evening Debbie collapsed in the bathroom in the foster home. An empty bottle of aspirins was found, and Debbie was rushed to the hospital. She told the psychiatrist who saw her the following day that she wished "to end it all" and had swallowed the aspirins "on purpose" (all eight of them!).

At that juncture she was returned to her foster home and arrangements were made to have her examined at the out-patient psychiatric department of the local hospital. However, Debbie failed to keep her appointment. In company with another girl from the foster home she hitchhiked to Vancouver. According to police reports, Debbie was picked up in Sudbury, Ontario by three older youths who drove her and her friend to Vancouver. She was reported to the police when she attended the emergency ward of a hospital for treatment of vaginal bleeding. She was in a rundown condition, and there was evidence of bruising on various parts of her body. She had neither money nor identification. A note on her medical file indicated that Debbie had made some superficial scratches on her wrist after being told she was being returned to Toronto.

Subsequently Debbie was placed in a group home in Hamilton, Ontario. During her first week in the home, one of the youths with whom Debbie had lived in Vancouver attempted to visit her. Because the staff smelled alcohol on his breath, his visit was forbidden. In response, Debbie broke some furniture in her room and the washroom mirror.

> She required nine stitches to repair two gashes which she opened on her right arm. Shortly after this incident Debbie ran away from the group home. Three days later she was picked up by the police in a bar in downtown Toronto.

The judge, in ordering her admittance to training school, noted his reluctance in taking such action but felt that Debbie required "close supervision for her own protection."

In the reception center Debbie quickly caught on to the routine and related well to the staff. She was very cautious in her interactions with the older girls in the unit but did develop friendships with two of the newer girls. There were only two negative reports on her file during her stay in reception. On one occasion she had broken a dining room rule by giving her dessert to another girl, and on another occasion she had to be placed in isolation to calm her down after an altercation with one of the older girls.

Reports from the institution's professional staff supported previous findings by concluding that there was no evidence of major psychopathology in Debbie's case, and no indications that Debbie would require a setting with maximum security features. The following statements are representative of the conclusions of the three-week assessment:

> Debbie's problems are of recent origin and likely are reactive to an unstable home situation.
>
> It is reasonable to conjecture that Debbie's recent antisocial behavior represents her overreaction to a number of situational, environmental and personal stresses which have unfortunately occurred simultaneously. (The report noted the transfer to a new school, the uncertainty of her parent's relationships, her awakening sexual interest, her choice of companions and her scholastic failure.)
>
> Debbie's self-esteem has suffered considerable damage in recent months and it is clear that basically she is an intelligent, thoughtful, sensitive girl who requires a period of time in a sheltered environment free from the stresses of her home life to enable her to consolidate her potentialities. It would be helpful to involve Debbie in counseling related to her sexual identity and to attempt to involve her in family therapy in order to reduce the present conflict with her mother.

The supervisors (matrons) reported that although Debbie related well to the staff and girls they felt more time was required for an adequate assessment because "we haven't seen the real Debbie yet."

The file was examined by the institution's psychiatrist who saw no reason to differ with the earlier diagnosis of adjustment reaction of adolescence. Psychiatric intervention was not considered to be necessary.

Debbie was transferred to another training school which provided academic training appropriate to her high academic potential.

Within a month Debbie absconded from the institution in company with two of her friends. They were apprehended within an hour while hitchhiking on the highway several hundred yards from the institution.

In accordance with the institution's regulations, the girls were placed in isolation on return to the school. While in isolation the girls spent their time banging on the doors, screaming at the top of their lungs, and cursing the institution and all of its staff. On the second day the school nurse was summoned to examine the girls when they were found smearing the walls of their rooms with blood. They had apparently chipped plaster off the walls and used it to cut their arms. The nurse reported that the wounds were superficial scratches and required only gauze bandages. Debbie had cut her arm in four places and had scratched on her left forearm the words *hate* and *love*.

The girls were subsequently separated to prevent them from influencing each other again. It was thought that Debbie had been the instigator of the cutting episode. She was returned to the reception center for transfer to a maximum security unit. In this unit she quickly developed a close relationship with one of the supervisors who she called her "training school mom." Three weeks later Debbie was caught twice in one day out of bounds. She had left her ward without permission and gone to visit this woman who was temporarily working on another ward. As a punishment she was required to forfeit television for one week and was forbidden to visit her training school mom. That evening while confined to her room she used a needle to cut on her left thigh in scratchy lettering: *To Mom with all my Hate*.

When the cuts were discovered, Debbie was again confined to her room. She spent hours just sitting on the bare floor rhythmically rocking back and forth and intermittently shouting and screaming. She screamed so much that she lost her voice. That evening she ripped her clothing and her bedsheets, and when the staff attempted to calm her down she threw her food tray at them and smeared food over the walls of her room. Her privileges were suspended indefinitely.

During her third week in the maximum security unit Debbie was involved in what the girls called a "lightbulb party." This involved a group of four girls who smashed a light bulb and then used the glass to lacerate their skin. Debbie cut herself on her thighs and breasts. Her cuts were long and quite deep but did not require stitches. They were grossly disfiguring and in the opinion of the institution's medical staff the scars were likely to be permanent.

The girls were placed in dissociation cells where they remained for three days. On the second day Debbie was taken for an interview with the psychiatrist when the staff found a note in her room in which she talked of hanging herself with a bedsheet. It was the psychiatrist's view that she was not a suicide risk and that her previous suicide gesture (with aspirins) was not a serious suicide attempt. However, he recommended that she be immediately involved in psychotherapy.

His report confirmed earlier diagnostic impressions and pointed out that Debbie was intelligent, articulate, and insightful, had no impairment of thinking, and displayed appropriate affect and good reality contact. Her behavioral deterioration was seen as partly manipulative and defiant (limit testing) and partly reactive to situational stress and encouragement from negative peers. Close supervision was recommended, and staff were asked to be supportive but firm in dealing with her.

At a case conference it was determined that Debbie should be seen for intensive psychotherapy by a member of the psychology staff. Arrangements were also made to have her separated from the group of girls with whom she had been associating. Her parents were asked to attend counseling sessions.

She was seen twice a week by her therapist, to whom she became attached. She also developed a close relationship with one of the students from the nearby university who visited Debbie as a volunteer counselor. However, less than two weeks after psychotherapy began, Debbie drank a "glass cocktail"–she ground up glass from a broken window into fine crystals and swallowed them in a glass of water. She was treated in the emergency ward of the local hospital and then transferred to the adolescent ward of a psychiatric hospital for observation.

The evaluation from the psychiatric hospital concluded that Debbie's needs would be best served by returning her to training school and arranging for her to be involved in summer school. The report stressed the fact that Debbie had related well to her therapist at the training school and that her problems were not those for which the program at the hospital's adolescent unit were designed. They further noted the absence of psychoneutrotic symptomatology and supported the previous findings of Adolescent Adjustment Reaction. Comment was made about Debbie's negative influence on other patients and on her need for treatment in a controlled environment.

Debbie was extremely bitter about her return to the training school. She had enjoyed her brief stay at the hospital, particularly because it was coeducational and she had many privileges not available at the training school–particularly smoking. Three days after returning to the school she attempted to escape in company with another girl, and when placed in detention following her capture, she slashed her left wrist with wire which she had pried off the mesh grill on the door. The laceration required several stitches. Debbie removed the stitches several hours after they were inserted. Accordingly the medical staff restitched the wound and covered her left arm in a plaster cast. While waiting in the emergency ward after the cast had been put on, Debbie took a wire coat hanger from a cupboard, broke it in half, and hid it in the cast. Later that evening she broke open the cast, once more removed the stitches, and then lacerated her right wrist and cut her thighs. She was summarily returned to the psychiatric hospital.

Although the staff were suspicious that she was manipulating and encouraging other patients to act-out, during her initial period in the hospital, Debbie personally presented no major problems. Family therapy had been suggested on admission, and Debbie's mother and father were relating well both to one another and to Debbie. Debbie seemed somewhat indifferent about her parents' newly established relationship, but she was elated when the staff informed her that she would soon be able to spend a weekend at home. Three days before the scheduled weekend visit she burned herself with a cigarette on her legs, stomach, and face. Two other patients who were known to be her friends also burned themselves. Debbie refused to discuss the incident. Debbie's weekend visit was cancelled. She immediately absconded with two male patients from the adolescent unit.

It was later related that she left her companions the following day after spending the night in a downtown garage. She proceeded to hitchhike to Toronto where she met some former training school girls in the downtown area. The girls had rented a luxury apartment, the rent of which they paid by prostituting and distributing drugs. Debbie denied having been involved in their prostitution activity. However, she appeared to have indulged heavily in alcohol and drugs. Seven days after she arrived she was rushed to the emergency unit of a Toronto hospital in a convulsive state after having ingested a large number of gravol pills in an attempt to "come down" off an amphetamine-induced high. When she was well enough Debbie was returned to the psychiatric hospital.

There she was placed on a locked ward rather than in the adolescent unit. Attempts were made to involve her in the milieu therapy program and in occucutional therapy. She was also assigned to a female therapist who had had considerable experience working with acting-out adolescents. Debbie's response was satisfactory for several weeks, but she then regressed after she was counseled when suspected of manipulating other patients into giving her cigarettes. She was reported to have exposed herself to several male patients in exchange for their phenobarbital and other medication. In addition she absconded while on an outing and was arrested for soliciting. Following her return to the hospital she broke several windows and threw light bulbs at fellow patients. Subsequently returned once more to the training school's maximum secuirty unit, she cut varous parts of her body on fourteen occasions in the first two weeks.

While on a downtown shopping trip which she earned through good behavior, she attempted to abscond. She was apprehended and returned to the institution where her negative behavior was punished by loss of offgrounds privileges. Her reaction was dramatic—using the metal clasp on her brassiere she cut an elaborate design on her stomach. A week later she was rushed to the hospital having been reported to have swallowed cleaning fluid which she had stolen from the staff cupboard. There was some doubt that she had actually done so. On three occasions in the next month she lacerated her hands by pushing them through windows.

Debbie had cut herself a total of twenty-three times since her first appearance in juvenile court. The cuts varied from about one inch to eight inches in length. She also had some superficial scratches and rudimentary tatoos. The twenty-three cuts were sufficiently deep to be both disfiguring and permanent. She also had nine scars on various parts of her body caused by self-inflicted burns and other injuries. No reports were available on the damage she had done to herself internally through swallowing glass and other foreign objects.

1 Introduction

More than a decade ago a group of clinical psychologists from the University of Waterloo were asked to provide clinical and research services at a training school for delinquent girls in a small town in Ontario, Canada. The training school, Grandview School, was an institution for twelve- to seventeen-year-old adolescent girls who had been admitted to the institution following a long history of delinquent behavior. Truancy, alcohol and drug abuse, theft, vandalism, prostitution, assault, extreme and chronic disruptive behavior in school and at home were characteristic behaviors in the backgrounds of these adolescents. Many of the girls had previously presented serious management problems in other institutional and community settings. This institution, we were to learn, was considered by many officials as the final measure available to cope with these girls. They were the failures of the juvenile justice system.

The Setting

The names of correctional institutions are often deceptively gentle. Millhaven, Oak Ridges, Collins Bay, White Oaks, Kawartha Lakes—all serve to convey a sense of serenity which stands in absurd contrast to their institutional function. It is a particularly peculiar twist of human thought that enables us to associate such benign terms with the structures we build to incarcerate our adult offenders and our delinquents.

Custody, security, discipline, deprivation, regimentation, isolation, repression, deterrence, and stigmatization are the institutional functions which such names fail to convey or intentionally conceal. Euphemism, irony and paradox abound in corrections. Grandview was no exception.

To the casual observer it seemed to be an idyllic setting. It had the appearance of a wealthy private girl's school. It was located on the periphery of a small town in Ontario. Nestled in a wooded glade, enriched by grassy fields, it bore not a single exterior trapping of detention or restraint. There were no towers, no ominous concrete, brick, or mortar walls, no barbed wire, or patrolling guards. A sign at the entrance announced its purpose in sedate curlicue—School for Girls. The few fences in evidence would be considered commonplace in any public school. Visitors repeatedly confused the local high school with the manicured lawns and unassuming buildings of Grandview, the training school. There was a singular, stark exception: a building not easily seen by the casual observer. All attempts to have this structure blend into the otherwise gentle surrounds were to prove futile. This was the maximum security unit which confined thirty-two intractable twelve- to sixteen-year-old girls in an oppressive atmosphere of locked doors, wire-mesh-grilled windows, steel bars, and cells.

First Impressions

When we first arrived at Grandview we were horrified by many things. It had a distinct and persistent military ambience. Discipline, we were told, was of paramount concern, and second only to custody. We were appalled at what we saw: the drab uniforms that the girls wore, the dull battleship gray or institutional green of the interior walls, the sterility and barreness of the girls' rooms, and teenage girls forced to march from place to place. The adolescents spent their evenings sitting around a large common room, in alphabetical order, in silence, knitting or crocheting or staring off into space, or simply chewing their nails or screwing up their faces trying not to cry, or just hanging their heads in boredom or depression (speaking was forbidden, crying was punished). Even the passing of secret messages by an elaborate gestural language that the ever vigilant matrons could never understand provided only transient relief from the oppressive atmosphere. This was discipline in its most Dickensian sense; discipline fashioned after some distorted Victorian notion that persisted in the program, in the selection of personnel, in the innumerable rules and regulations, and even in the rather quaint practice of naming the buildings after famous British naval figures such as Nelson, Drake, and Collingwood.

We were dismayed by the sight of teenagers locked up in concrete and steel cells; by matrons carrying large rings of huge, dangling brass keys; by the solitary confinement units; by the horsehair mattresses; by beds welded to the floors; by the omnipresent tension that permeated the atmosphere.

The appearance of the girls was a source of considerable concern. They were often grossly obese or emaciated, shabbily dressed, pale from lack of makeup or exposure to the sun, disheveled and unkempt. What concerned us most was the fact that many of them, most of them in fact, were scarred.

Carving

Almost every girl had ugly cuts and scars on her legs, her hands, and her arms. Some had scars that looked like initials or hearts or swastikas on their faces. Not tattoos. Not nicely colored decorative designs, although some had these too. These were cuts; gouges in their skin. Otherwise attractive, pretty teenagers grossly disfigured by permanent lesions. Some girls were literally covered with scars.

We quickly learned that these cuts were self-inflicted. The girls, as they put it, had *carved* themselves. It was an apt choice of terms; an operational term for a behavior analogous to carving a roast. They had deliberately sliced their skin. The cuts were sufficiently deep to ensure permanent scarring. They had used needles, nail files, steel-edged rulers or anything else you might image, such as plaster chipped off the walls, or pens or pencils, or broken glass or china, or utensils smuggled from the dining room, or pins stolen from the sewing room. They also used instruments you might not imagine such as wood splinters from tables and chairs, nails pried out of furniture or shoes, food bones, metal ends of shoe laces, broken eye glasses, toothpaste tubes, and dentures. If nothing else was available they would pull out a strand of their hair and use it as a saw, or break off their fingernails or toenails and use them as knives. Enterprising young ladies.

When the university began its affiliation with the training school there were 136 girls in the institution, 117 had carved at least once. Eighty-six percent of the population had mutilated themselves. Many girls had carved themselves on multiple occasions. The average girl had lacerated her skin eight times. The same figures describe almost any period in the thirty or so years of the institution's history. It was a perennial problem.

We also learned that many of the girls had swallowed pins or had inserted needles under their skin. Some girls had deliberately burned themselves by means of cigarettes, matches, hot objects, or scalding substances. Some had scarred themselves by rubbing their bodies with or against some rough object. Some girls had broken windows, crushed the glass, and then, filling their hands with water, had drunk the glass chips. They referred to this as their "glass cocktail." They had, in fact, swallowed a startling array of things from combs to cleaning fluids.

The girls' self-mutilatory behavior had continued throughout the years in spite of the best efforts of the staff to control it. Security measures were of little value—the girls were much too enterprising. Their ingenuity was boundless. Girls who had been stripped, searched, and placed in a solitary confinement cell (variously and euphemistically referred to as a "dissociation unit," "thinking room," "blue room," "cooling off room") with little else than a hospital style nightgown and a mattress would frequently and consistently astound the staff by managing to mutilate themselves.

We found that self-mutilators had been counseled, punished, lectured, cajoled, reprimanded, educated, and isolated—all to no avail. The staff had made them hide their scars by wearing extra clothing. They had punished them for carving by reducing the limited number of privileges which they had, or by disallowing visitors, or by assigning extra work, or by delaying their release from the institution. If there is any substance to the reports communicated to us, at one point in the institution's history a standard treatment of carving was the application of salt directly to the wound with a toothbrush!

The staff's punishing techniques were as innovative and as varied as the girls' techniques for mutilating themselves. All of the staff's corrective measures were impressively unsuccessful. The behavior persisted, at times it worsened.

The matrons developed considerable expertise in assessing the extent of wounds and were consistently successful at predicting the number of sutures required for a wound. Local physicians were engaged in a shuttle service from their offices to the local hospital for wound stitching or stomach pumping. The stitches were often removed by the girls shortly after they were applied.

In addition to our own efforts to treat and understand the girls' self-destructive behavior, the resources of a major university were brought to bear on the problem. Through the largesse of a major funding agency, financial support was made readily available. The facilities, personnel, and resources of the Ontario government's correctional services branch were provided to support, augment, and encourage these efforts. Despite this, the behavior persisted.

Psychiatrists, social workers, criminologists, psychiatric nurses, recreational therapists, priests, ministers, and psychologists attempted to treat the girls through a wide variety of intervention techniques. Volunteers were recruited from high schools, colleges, universities, local nurses' residences, and church groups to arrange activites, to play with the girls, and to treat them. Pastoral counselors, clinical psychology interns, and student social workers with empathy and enthusiasm tried to help the girls.

Individual psychotherapy was tried, as was psychodrama, art therapy, music therapy, milieu therapy, group psychotherapy, relaxation therapy, behavior therapy (covert conditioning, contingency management, token economy), family therapy, educational therapy, and sensitivity training. Major improvements were made in the institutional environment. The decor was improved, the rules were relaxed, the community was involved, the staff were trained, the "sentences" shortened, the privileges broadened. The self-mutilation persisted.

Better-educated staff were hired. Male staff were recruited. Close to a hundred volunteers from local universities were introduced. Probably the best inmate to staff ratio that ever existed in such institutions was achieved. Available to the girls were a large number of helpers ranging from the local ladies auxiliary to clinical psychologists of international renown.

The behavior persisted, at times it worsened.

We found ourselves providing crisis service twenty-four hours a day. Visits to the local hospital emergency wards became routine. We observed the girls' behavior, interviewed the staff and girls, held case conferences, surveyed the literature, corresponded with experts on self-mutilation, brainstormed, introspected, interviewed parents, and sought advice from administrators in other institutions. We tried every conceivable treatment that held any promise.

Over the years we were alternately elated and depressed. We experienced short periods of enthusiasm, when we would become encouraged by the rationality and promise of a new approach. This would be followed by periods when we lapsed into self-recrimination, frustration, and cynicism as we faced the reality of the abject failure of our best efforts and the shortcomings of the most sophisticated therapies. Our most frequent response was anger. Frustrated by our efforts we attributed the responsibility for these failures to anything which we perceived as blocking our efforts. Rather than accepting the importance of the treatment as the reason for our failure, we explained it by questioning the competence of our staff, the cooperation of the administration, the oppression of the environment, the management strategies of the directors, and even the opposition of co-workers in other disciplines. Sometimes our blaming was appropriate; sometimes it was unrealistic; always it was useless. There was no one whom we did not at some point come to view as the source of our frustration. Most of the time, however, we fully realized that all of the staff shared our concern for alleviating the distress of these girls and for controlling and preventing their self-mutilating behavior. Of course, we also questioned the validity of the total juvenile correctional system and our participation in it. Vast social system change was well beyond our energies, capabilities, vision, and patience. The problem was immediate and, we stubbornly believed, solvable.

We even blamed the girls for their failure to respond to our treatment. We had tried to humanize their environment. We were making available to them the best treatments that social and medical science had to offer. In return they gave us crises, demands, complaints, belligerence, insults, belittlement, rejection—and blood. Why would they not cooperate?

Gradually we learned. We learned by the mistakes we made; we learned by being forced to confront our naivete; we learned from the failure of traditional therapies; we learned from years of frustration; we learned from what our associates viewed as stubborn persistence; we learned through desperation. Mostly we learned by the humility that was forced upon us by the negative outcomes of our finest professional efforts. We learned only after we were willing to concede that we did not understand the girls' behavior, when we suspended our clinical judgment, when we grudgingly allowed the girls to explain their behavior to us, and when we stopped playing expert and allowed ourselves to become students. The girls became our teachers. As students we were slow learners, but what the girls told us finally sank through our professional biases and misconceptions. Not only did the girls teach us how to understand their self-mutilatory behavior, but they also led us to the development of an intervention technique which enabled them to eliminate self-mutilation in the institution in the space of a few weeks from the inception of *their program*. The girls led us to develop an unorthodox strategy for the control and prevention of at least one form of self-mutilation. This strategy may have potential as a model for understanding and treating many other forms of self-mutilatory behavior.

The treatment program will be described in subsequent chapters of this book. We feel that the program attests to the value of listening to adolescents rather than reacting to them.

The program is also testimony to the value of a field-theoretical or grounded theory approach to social science research. We had been impressed, negatively, by the fact that, in corrections, treatment programs are typically adopted and promulgated not on the basis of evidence of their efficacy but on the basis of their promise. Only rarely are programs subjected to the kind of evaluation process which would allow one to assess whether they help or harm. Correctional programs are often adopted on the basis of impression, appearance, packaging, novelty, or popularity. In the search for panaceas a multitude of inappropriate programs have been employed and later discarded (Ross and Price, 1976; Ross, 1977; Ross and McKay, 1978a; Gendreau and Ross, 1979).

At the outset of our search for a solution to carving, we determined that we wished to provide continual evaluation of any and all programs we tried. We would continue or discard programs not on the basis of popularity or impressions or heuristic appeal but on the basis of objective evidence that they were or were not effective. The effects of our treatment would be subjected to continual scrutiny. Programs which did not prove worthwhile would be dropped.

Our sequential research strategy enabled us to obtain information at each stage of the project on the basis of which we could introduce improvements to our programs for new groups of girls entering our treatment units. This was a long-term multistage project in which programs in each stage were conceptualized on the basis of the results of previous phases and, in turn, yielded hypotheses for treatment in subsequent stages.

The Riddle

In this book we present a riddle. During our research project we eliminated self-mutilation three times:

1. The first time we did not know we had eliminated self-mutilation, let alone how we had done so.
2. The second time we knew we had eliminated self-mutilation, but we did not know how.
3. The third time self-mutilation was eliminated was when we deliberately and systematically employed the rather unorthodox strategies which we had unwittingly used the first two times.

Our intervention strategy is based on an unorthodox conceptualization of self-mutilatory behavior which we will describe in chapter 8. It is a view with which many might quarrel. It is the only conceptualization of self-mutilatory behavior which for us makes sense out of the observations, ironies, contradictions, experiences, and data we collected in our long-term research project. But it is disconcertingly uncomplicated and clearly conjectural. It amounts to little more than a hypothesis which we arrived at as a means of making sense out of our experience. It represents only one alternative to a host of far more sophisticated and elegant interpretations and explanations of self-mutilation which we found in the literature. These we found wanting in terms of their value in suggesting treatment techniques which might ameliorate carving in our population of self-mutilators. However, it is essential that the reader evaluate the adequacy of our explanation of carving in relation to the wide variety of explanations of other forms of self-mutilation. It is our view that our conceptualization of carving might be useful as a way of viewing other forms of self-injurious behavior.

In chapter 3 we provide a report of the prevalence and forms of self-mutilation in other settings in order to provide a broader perspective within which to view the carving of our subjects. As we shall see, self-mutilation is by no means an uncommon phenomenon. It is not limited to institutional settings or to psychiatric or correctional populations. The variety of forms of self-mutilation is almost endless, limited only by the imagination of the mutilator. Equally varied are the explanations of self-mutilation which are discussed in chapter 4.

One characteristic of self-mutilation on which almost every investigator agrees is its remarkable resistance to treatment. The types of therapeutic and management techniques which have been applied to control self-mutilators are critically discussed and evaluated in chapter 5.

Our own treatment-research program is described in chapters 6, 7, and 8. A descriptive study of carving at Grandview is presented in chapter 6. Chapter 7 details our treatment efforts with the adolescent self-mutilators at Grandview. Chapter 8 presents a reappraisal of our treatment efforts and describes the development of an intervention approach, "co-opting," which led to the elimination of carving at Grandview.

2 The Scope of Self-Mutilation

It appears that a common characteristic of training schools, perhaps of correctional institutions in general, is that they are crisis oriented. When the staff are not occupied with responding to a crisis they tend to be preoccupied with anticipating one. Grandview was no exception. Incidents of self-mutilation were by no means the only type of crises with which the staff were forced to cope. Assaults, abscondance, vandalism, and fighting were everyday occurrences. The girls had an incredible proclivity for horseplay, manipulation, theft, property destruction, homosexual activity, disruption, and histrionics. At any particular moment it was not unusual for the staff on one ward to be cleaning up the debris left by a girl who had, in a fit of rage, shattered the furniture in her room, while the staff on an adjacent ward were cleaning up the room of another girl who had smeared the walls with her blood; or were chasing a group of girls who were running pell mell down the hill in an abortive or successful attempt at escape; or were struggling to cut off the water supply to the room of another girl who had flooded the ward by continually flushing her toilet, the bowl of which she had plugged with clothes and paper; or were trying to console a hysterical girl who had just been told that her mother could not make it for her visit, again.

Because we had, perhaps unwisely, accepted a major share of the responsibility for providing treatment for these girls, we were obliged to respond immediately to these crises wherever and whenever they occurred. We were on call twenty-four hours a day, seven days a week for several years. We were literally engulfed by the place.

Our total involvement in the institution narrowed our vision. It led to our perceiving the self-mutilatory behavior of these adolescent girls as a unique local phenomenon. We tended to think that it was a behavior which was peculiar to adolescent girls and, specifically, adolescent girls in correctional institutions. Our perception was reinforced by the literature we obtained which contained many reports of self-cutting behavior in other similar institutions both in North America and Britain—reports that often fostered the view that such behavior is to be found almost exclusively with girls. It was only after we became more familiar with the broader literature on self-injurious behavior that we were able to obtain a balanced perspective of the self-mutilation of the girls at Grandview. Self-mutilatory behavior was by no means endemic to our setting, or to institutions for adolescent girls. It is not an isolated phenomenon which is to be found only in girls, or only in institutions, or only among disturbed delinquents. It is a very commonly occurring phenomenon of major and increasing social significance.

To list the variety of ways in which humans have contrived, for whatever reason, to produce physical injury or damage to their own bodies is to give testimony to their ingenuity, if not their perversity. Humans have lacerated themselves, poisoned themselves, burned themselves, gassed themselves, blinded themselves, severed their limbs, and swallowed impressively indigestible objects ranging from needles to faucet handles.

Humans have demonstrated a remarkable capacity to inflict injury upon themselves by deliberate falling, pounding parts of their body, hitting, ripping, slapping, jabbing themselves, and inserting objects under their skin. They have rubbed, sucked, and licked raw the skin on various parts of their body. They have chewed their nails, their fingers, their lips. They have removed their own nails, amputated their fingers and toes, pulled out their hair, sewn up their mouths, severed their Achilles tendons, disembowelled themselves, and even plucked out their eyes.

The effects of such self-injurious behavior have been equally varied. Self-mutilators have permanently disfigured their appearance with welts, bruises, gouges, gashes, and lacerations. Permanent neurological damage has been effected by self-injurious behaviors such as head banging or inhalation of gas. Kidney and other internal organ damage has been achieved by ingestion of various chemicals. Permanent skin damage has resulted from burning. Fingers and toes have been lost through self-amputation. Sexual incapacity has resulted from castration and other forms of genital self-mutilation. Retinas have been dislodged by head banging, eye gouging, and eye poking. A wide variety of skin disorders have resulted from rubbing, scouring, and scalding. Limbs have been broken and severed.

For reasons which are not altogether clear, such self-mutilating behaviors often occur in the absence of any reported discomfort or pain. The absence of discomfort, however, does not extend to the parents or friends of self-mutilators. It is the rare individual who fails to be distressed by the sight of the mutilated patient or who fails to be repulsed by the apparently senseless gashing, ripping, or tearing of flesh, or the amputations, or burning of the self-mutilator. Even after years of exposure to physical trauma, case-hardened attendants, including medical staff, still react with revulsion to many of the insults to the bodies of self-mutilating patients. The reaction is perhaps most pronounced in those who have responsibility for the individual, such as caseworkers, attendants, medical staff, or parents. The reaction to a bloodied, burned, scarred, damaged individual is frequently a mixture of revulsion and guilt. No less common are reactions of frustration, incredibility, and outright anger at the apparently nonsensical assault that the person has made on his body.

At the risk of appearing callous we must mention that there are also serious effects in economic terms. Many self-mutilators persist for years in their attacks on their bodies and repeatedly present themselves or are presented to emergency wards, general hospitals, and psychiatric centers. Frequently, in institutional settings such patients require individual supervision on a round-the-clock basis. They require intervention by medical doctors, psychiatrists, dermatologists, psychologists, and plastic surgeons. These patients present major concerns and financial burdens to workmen's compensation boards, unemployment insurance agencies, and general insurance companies who are becoming more and more concerned about costs of treating the self-inflicted injuries of these individuals. Many insurance companies have employed special investigators to deal with such matters. Police are often required to respond to incidents of citizen injury only to discover (or suspect) after time-consuming investigation that the injury was self-inflicted. Such "public mischief" cases appear to be increasingly common. But clearly of greatest concern is the fact that the damage that the mutilator does to himself, often under transient conditions of stress, remains long after the stress has gone—he remains mutilated for life.

It would be reassuring to most of us if self-mutilation represented only the bizarre reaction of a small number of deranged individuals carefully sequestered out of the public eye in the back wards of some institution for the psychiatrically ill. As we shall see, such is not the case. Self-mutilation is not exclusively found in institutional settings, nor is it restricted to severely disturbed individuals. Just as there is no part of the human body which has not been mutilated, there is no setting where self-mutilation has not occurred. Self-injury has been reported as an everyday occurrence in settings housing retarded or autistic children. Correctional institutions for adult offenders frequently have to cope with inmates who injure themselves. Epidemics of self-mutilation have been reported in such institutions and are commonplace in many correctional settings for juvenile delinquents. Incidents of self-mutilation have been reported in detention centers, receiving homes, group foster homes, university residences, infant daycare centers, and facilities for senior citizens.

In contrast to the myth, it is by no means only adolescent females who indulge in such behavior; it is frequently found in both males and females of all ages ranging from five months to old age. Nor is it exclusively the behavior of deranged or defective individuals lacking an adequate grasp of reality or an inadequate appreciation of the consequences of their acts. It has been reported in normal, rational, cortically intact individuals, in apparently healthy infants, and even in animals.

Self-mutilation of various sorts has been reported as socially acceptable behavior in various cultural groups. The anthropological literature is replete with examples of initiation ceremonies involving self-mutilatory behavior such as teeth filing, nose piercing, feet binding, and breast removal.

The methods used by self-mutilators are as varied as the forms that their bodily injury has taken. They have cut themselves with knives, razors, scissors, and an endless variety of other objects. They have swallowed glass, bleach, stones, needles, solvents, lighter fluid, nails, wire, spoons and knives. They have slapped, punched, and kicked themselves and beat, pounded, and hurled their bodies against objects. They have poked their eyes, stuck fingers in doors, and deliberately fallen down stairs. They have induced seizures. Innumerable objects such as needles and pins, paper clips, nails, combs, and knives have been inserted under the skin or in bodily orifices. Self-mutilators have walked on hot coals and on glass and have burned themselves with matches and cigarettes and stuck their fingers into electric outlets. They have deliberately refused or interfered with essential medical treatment, refused to eat, removed sutures, and destroyed plaster casts protecting broken limbs. Some enterprising self-mutilators have given themselves frostbite by urinating on their toes and then deliberately putting their feet out of windows in below-zero weather. There have been recent case reports of self-trepanning in which the mutilator used an electric drill to open a hole in her head. Individuals have severely damaged themselves in apparent abortion attempts using numerous means including dashing themselves against sharp objects, consuming various dangerous substances, deliberately falling down stairs, or shooting themselves in the abdomen.

There is little agreement as to the appropriate method of prevention or treatment of self-mutilation or the explanation of such behavior. In part this is because self-mutilation encompasses a wide variety of topographically distinct behaviors performed by heterogeneous populations in an equally varied number of settings employing diverse methods of injuring themselves and apparently for many different reasons. It is also attributable to the fact that self-mutilation comes under the purview of many disciplines which tend to approach it from often radically different perspectives.

The literature on self-mutilation is voluminous. Reports of cases, epidemiological surveys, descriptions of treatment programs and research reports appear in widely scattered sources. Attempting to make sense, or even order, out of this vast literature is a formidable task.

In addition, the search for an explanation of such behaviors has been greatly hampered by definitional problems. Investigators have used myriad terms in reference to self-mutilatory behaviors, and it is seldom the case that the same term refers to the same behaviors. The converse is also true. A specific form of self-mutilatory behavior is referred to by many labels by different investigators. Classification, the building block of science, is at its most primitive level in the study of self-mutilation.

Equally troubling is the fact that many investigators seem to fail to realize the breadth of behaviors which can be subsumed under the category of self-mutilation. As a result they operate in an experimental vacuum and are apparently unaware of the investigations of others. Accordingly their explanations of the behavior and their suggestions for treatment are highly circumscribed. We are a long way from the kind of integration of ideas and concepts and cross-fertilization that might lead to a breakthrough in our understanding of self-mutilatory behavior.

Table 2-1
Self-mutilatory Behavior: Illustrative Terms

1. A little suicide	17. Self-assaultive behavior
2. Attempted suicide	18. Self-attacking behavior
3. Attenuated suicide	19. Self-damaging behavior
4. Autoaggression	20. Self-destructive behavior
5. Deliberate disability	21. Self-harming behavior
6. Deliberate self-harm	22. Self-hurting behavior
7. Deliberate self-injury	23. Self-injurious behavior
8. Demonstrative self-injury	24. Self-poisoning behavior
9. Focal suicide	25. Self-punitive behavior
10. Intentional injury	26. Self-stimulatory behavior
11. Local self-destruction	27. Self-wounding behavior
12. Malingering	28. Self-directed aggression
13. Masochism	29. Self-mutilation
14. Munchausen syndrome	30. Small suicide
15. Self-abusive behavior (or conduct)	31. Symbolic wounding
	32. Parasuicide
16. Self-aggressive behavior	33. Purposive accidents

Table 2-1 illustrates the wide variety of terms that have been used by investigators to refer to self-mutilatory behavior. It is not uncommon in the literature to find many of these employed in a single report. However, there appears to be some preference among investigators for at least three terms: *self-injurious behavior* (Azrin et al., 1975; Bachman, 1972; Ballinger, 1971; Bancroft et al., 1975; Baroff, 1976; Cautela and Baron, 1973; Cookson, 1977; Corte, Wolff, and Locke, 1971; Duker, 1975; Fielding and Cole, 1971; Harris and Raik, 1976; Lucero et al., 1976; Matthews, 1968; Mishara, Robertson, and Kastenbaum, 1973; Money, Wolff, and Annecillo, 1972; Morrison, 1972; Myers, 1975; Repp and Deitz, 1974; Romanczyk and Goren, 1975; Sandow, 1975; Schaefer, 1970; Simpson, 1975; Singh, 1976; Skrimshire, 1976; Smolev, 1971; Tanner and Zeiler, 1975; Tate, 1972; Weiher, 1975; Whitehead and Ferrence, 1973a,b; Williams, 1974); *self-mutilation* (Bach-Y-Rita, 1974; Bergman, 1975; Burnham, 1969; Claghorn and Beto, 1967; Clanon, 1965; Cooper and Fowlie, 1973; Crabtree and Grossman, 1974; Davidson, 1962; French and Nelson, 1972; Gardner and Gardner, 1975; Goldney and Simpson, 1975; Green, 1968; Johnson, 1973; Kafka, 1969; Korten et al., 1975; Lester, 1972; Lester and Lester, 1971; McKerracher, Loughane and Watson, 1968; Miller and Bashkin, 1974; Mutter et al., 1975; Offer and Barlow, 1960; Panton, 1962; Podvoll, 1969; Ragain and Anson, 1976; Roback et al., 1972; Ryback, 1971; Shodell and Reiter, 1968; Simpson, 1973; Slawson and Davidson, 1964; Stinnett and Hollender, 1970; Virkkunen, 1976); and *self-destructive behavior* (Ferrence and Johnson, 1974; Green, 1968; Jones, Simmons, and Frankel, 1974; Lovaas and Simmons, 1969; Martin and Treffry, 1970; Merbaum, 1973; Peterson and Peterson, 1968; Saposnek and Watson, 1974; Varga, 1971; Wilbur, Chandler, and Carpenter, 1974).

It should be noted that some terms are more explanatory than descriptive (for example, *masochism; auto-aggression, self-attacking behavior*). They do little beyond identifying the theoretical orientation of the investigator. Such terms are frequently employed by investigators who subscribe to the popular view that the individual who harms himself is essentially redirecting aggressive impulses toward himself that, for whatever reason, he cannot direct outwardly against the person or object causing the aggressive impulse (Bachman, 1972; Marks, Rachman, and Gelder, 1965; Sandler, 1964; Tate and Baroff, 1966). Self-mutilation is aggression turned inward. Regardless of the adequacy of such an explanation these terms fail to identify the phenomenon to which the explanation applies. Furthermore, they create the problem that we cannot label behaviors as self-attacking unless we first assure ourselves by investigation that they, in fact, represent displaced aggression. Accordingly, classification must be made on the basis of explanation. The cart is put before the horse. Finally, such labels tend to reduce rather than augment effort in searching for explanations since the explanation is in effect forced by the label. The investigator tends, therefore, to view the behavior from a very narrow perspective and to expend effort in seeking evidence for, and sources of, aggression, rather than trying to understand the behavior. If the aggression-turned-inward hypothesis were satisfactory and did apply to all self-mutilatory behaviors, it would be appropriate to label these as auto-aggression or self-attacking. However, there are major shortcomings in the auto-aggression hypotheses (Lester, 1972). The adequacy and value of a classification scheme based on categories of explanation depends on the adequacy of the explanations. It is clear that the study of self-mutilation has by no means advanced to the point where we have developed adequate explanations of the phenomenon which would support an explanatory classification scheme.

Other terms (for example, *purposive accidents, deliberate or intentional injuries, malingering*) are used by investigators who are concerned with the manipulative or fraudulent aspects of self-mutilation. They are interested in those self-mutilators who intentionally injure themselves or simulate actual disease with the specific purpose of obtaining financial gain or other special compensation. As classificatory terms these labels share some of the shortcomings of other terms which imply explanation. In this instance the explanation is in terms of manipulation or intent rather than aggression (Atkins, 1978; Berkow, 1970; Hawkins, Jones, and Tibbetts, 1956). It is by no means a simple task to determine whether a specific act of self-mutilation is or is not intended to defraud. As Berkow (1970) has noted: "malingering is not a diagnosis, it is an accusation. To prove the charge requires detective work, not physical examination." To use these terms for classification or even identification is obviously problematic.

Terms such as *local self-destruction* and *small suicide*, remind us of the relationship between self-mutilation and suicide, a relationship which Menninger noted as eary as 1932. Menninger viewed self-mutilation as a suicidal act in which the suicidal impulse is directed to part of the body rather than to the whole body. Within his general classification of self-destructive behavior self-mutilation is referred to as *focal suicide*: suicidal impulses are focused on a part of the body which serves as a substitute for the whole body.

Menninger's scheme is one of the few systematic attempts to classify the wide variety of self-damaging behavior and is particularly valuable in pointing to the possibility of a relationship between self-mutilation, suicide, and other self-damaging behaviors such as smoking, alcohol and drug abuse, accident proneness, obesity, and the like. We prefer to avoid using the suicide or self-destructive model for classification of self-mutilation for several reasons.

Controversy has characterized the attempts of suicidologists at classification, and it would seem unwise to try to force self-mutilatory behavior into an already unsatisfactory schema. Doing so would complicate rather than clarify or simplify. Moreover, as Lester (1972) has pointed out, there is in the action of the self-mutilator seldom an intent to die and often very little risk of dying. Although the self-mutilator could engender his own death by his behavior, in the vast majority of cases this does not happen. His behavior is actually counter-intentional to suicide rather than suicidal. To view self-mutilation as a subtype or a variant of suicide is to encourage attempts to explain the behavior in terms of explanations of suicide. It is our view that to do so would impede progress in understanding self-mutilation since we simply do not know enough about the nature of the relationship between self-mutilation and suicide. In addition, little progress has been made in understanding the nature of the relationsip between self-mutilation and other forms of self-destructive behavior. It would seem advisable to investigate them separately before lumping them together within a particular conceptual framework.

After examining the wide literature on self-mutilation, we decided that it would be useful to adopt a behavioral-descriptive rather than an explanatory-based classification scheme. Such an approach makes it possible to at least approximate the classification stage of research. At the point of classification we wish to avoid the complexities and problems involved in attempting to examine the mutilator's motives or intentions or to determine the environmental or interpersonal conditions which may have preceded the act.

Table 2-2 presents our first approximation to a classification schema. Within our schema, self-mutilation is viewed as a particular form of a broader category of self-injurious behavior. Self-mutilation is differentiated from other self-injurious behaviors by virtue of the directness of the link between the behavior and its consequences. Whereas with overeating, smoking, or excessive ingestion of alcohol, the injury to the body may not be immediately apparent, in the case of self-mutilation the effects are immediate and direct.

In order to develop the subcategories of self-mutilation, we analyzed reports on hundreds of cases of self-mutilation which had been described in the literature. We determined that each of these could be subsumed under one of nine

Table 2-2
Classification

Self-injurious behaviors are: *Those measures carried out by the individual upon himself which tend to cut-off, to remove, to maim, to destroy, to render imperfect some part of the body.* —Philipps and Muzaffer (1961)

Direct Self-Injurious Behavior: Self-Mutilation	*Indirect Self-Injurious Behavior:*
The link between the behavior(s) and damaging consequence(s) to the body is temporally immediate and unequivocal.	The link between the behavior(s) and damaging consequence(s) to the body is temporally remote and equivocal.
Types Cutting Biting Abrading Severing Inserting Burning Ingesting or inhaling Hitting Constricting	Examples Obesity Alcohol abuse Smoking Drug abuse Glue sniffing Refusing medical treatment Maceration

categories of behavior: cutting, biting, abrading, severing, inserting, burning, ingesting or inhaling, hitting, and constricting. These categories allow one to classify most cases easily, objectively, and with a high degree of reliability. But the schema is not without shortcomings. For example, the categories are not entirely mutually exclusive. Furthermore, in many instances one must apply more than one category to a particular case because, quite frequently, an individual will mutilate himself in several ways during one episode. However, the classification scheme which we propose does serve us well in creating some order out of the mass of reports on self-mutilation, and it has the decided advantage of leaving both ourselves and our readers free to study direct self-injurious behavior unencumbered by theoretical biases derived from our understanding of suicide, alcoholism, obesity, and other indirect self-injurious behaviors. Such theories may or may not be useful to our attempts to understand direct self-injurious behavior, or self-mutilation. By subdividing direct self-injurious behaviors into more specific acts, we leave open the possibility that such behaviors not only are topographically or behaviorally distinct but also are unrelated functionally.

Clearly this classification allows us to further subdivide within each category on the basis of characteristics of the subjects (for example, age, sex, population) or setting (for example, psychiatric institution, correctional setting, community setting). There may, after all, be major and important motivational differences between, for example, the self-cutting of a chronically regressed schizophrenic adult patient in the back ward of a psychiatric hospital and the self-cutting of a socially alert adolescent girl in a correctional institution. Before lumping them together as though they were identical in all respects one should determine whether the same explanation can account for the behavior in the two different populations. At the present time there is simply no evidence which could justify our treating these as one.

It should also be noted that our choice of the present classification scheme is not in the least intended to reject the possibility of some kind of a link between self-mutilation and suicide. We merely feel that to try to identify that link is premature, given our present state of knowledge.

Within the proposed classification it is possible to subdivide the categories of self-mutilation in terms of the severity of the consequences. Within each category a continuum would exist from relatively minor damage at one extreme to death (that is, completed suicide) at the other extreme. Suicide may well be the outcome of a self-mutilating event even if it were not the intent.

We must admit to an overriding bias which prevailed on us in our seeking to leave open the possibility that the self-cutting of our adolescent subjects requires a different explanation than other forms of self-mutilation: our examination of the explanations provided by investigators of these other forms had profited us not at all in understanding or controlling the self-mutilation of our subjects.

3 Prevalence and Forms of Self-Mutilation

In this chapter we intend, by describing other forms of self-mutilation, to provide the reader with a broader perspective of the carving of our adolescent offenders.

Investigations and reports of self-mutilation are found in widely dispersed literature sources including anthropology, suicidology, criminology, psychiatry, psychology, dermatology, sociology, epidemiology, theology, psychoanalysis, and plastic surgery. In reviewing this literature we examined the abstracts in these fields, undertook literature searches through several computerized bibliographic retrieval services, and conducted a mail survey of key resource personnel and investigators. We also consulted with a large number of professionals who have had firsthand experience in coping with self-mutilators, plastic surgeons, general practitioners, emergency ward staff, psychiatrists, dermatologists, military personnel, anthropologists, staff in institutions for autistic and retarded children, offenders, and geriatric patients, and police officers.

It would be irresponsible of us not to caution you at this point that much of the material you will read is decidedly unpleasant. It can, we have learned from experience, have a substantial impact on the unsuspecting reader. We have learned this from the reactions of our own research staff, many of whom have had substantial field experience in correctional, psychiatric, and general hospital settings. We have observed strong reactions to this material from colleagues, students, clerical staff, and many others who have had occasion to become familiar with some of this literature. But most of all we have learned from our own reactions. We had accumulated considerable experience with the various forms of self-mutilation and had become inured to the ways in which individuals contrive to harm themselves. So we thought. In all candor we had underestimated the shock, horror and revulsion that are elicited when this behavior is described.

We have been and are concerned about the presentation of this type of material. It is difficult to avoid appearing sensational. As one of our colleagues with medical training reminded us when this issue was raised, the presentation of such material in accurate, descriptive, and objective style is essential if other investigators are to understand the precise nature and boundaries of the phenomenon. We thank him for this and concur. If you have a psychiatric or medical background and are familiar with such concrete descriptions, it is entirely possible that this material will not upset you. If you have not had this type of training our caution should be considered seriously in guiding your reading. On the other hand, we should note that there is a tendency for some investigators of self-mutilation to report their work in language devoid of affect. Although we understand this inclination, it can at times be misleading. Self-mutilation is a dramatic behavior. Clear understanding of the behavior can only be achieved, we believe, by conveying the affective context. It is necessary to constantly remind ourselves that the behavior, as it is described with all of the attendant affect and vivid description, is precisely that which practitioners confront in this field.

In presenting a review of the literature we have attempted to describe succinctly the forms which self-mutilation has taken. It is a voluminous literature. In order to illustrate the behaviors we have been deliberately selective, hopefully representative, and far from exhaustive.

Prevalence

In reviewing the literature on self-mutilation one is immediately impressed by statements as to its high frequency. Many of the following phrases are used: "quite common," "frequently," "prevalent," "well known." Data to support such statements are more difficult to find. This is partly because reports of the frequency of self-mutilation are buried within the data on broader categories of self-injury or suicide in such a way that one cannot extricate the information specific to self-mutilation. The problem is compounded by the fact that self-mutilatory behavior is referred to by such a wide variety of terms referring to such a heterogeneity of behaviors that one cannot ascertain what particular acts are included. Moreover, many reports fail to provide adequate information on the characteristics of the population from which samples are drawn, and in most instances we are unable to determine the representativeness of samples. Accordingly, it is not possible at the present time to provide even a reasonable guess as to the prevalence of self-mutilatory behavior, except in rather exceptional settings or population groupings. Considerable caution must be exercised in extrapolating from the data that are available.

In table 3-1 we present a summary of a number of selected studies which have provided some data relative to the prevalence of various self-mutilatory behaviors in an equally varied number of settings. The table is intended only to be illustrative.

We have included summaries of some large-scale epidemiological studies of the broader category of self-injurious behavior (which may or may not include suicide). The methodological problems involved in measuring the prevalence of self-injury are well documented in these studies (see particularly Whitehead and Ferrence, 1973a,b). These problems are compounded when one attempts to measure the incidence of a narrower category of self-injurious behavior such as self-mutilation. The epidemiological studies have focused attention on the phenomenon of self-injury by demonstrating the remarkable incidence of such behaviors—as high as 1,400 cases per annum per 100,000 population. (Whitehead and Ferrence, 1973 a,b). They have also demonstrated sex, occupation, education, age, socioeconomic, and geographic patterns in the incidence of self-injurious behaviors. We will not describe these patterns because it is our view that different patterns may well be found in the prevalence and distribution of self-mutilation as distinct from self-injury. Badly needed are epidemiological studies of self-mutilation of the quality of those conducted on self-injury by teams of researchers in Great Britain and in London, Ontario.

Table 3-1 makes it clear that the carving of the girls at Grandview was by no means an isolated phenomenon. It also shows that self-mutilation is not exclusively or predominantly a female problem. Nor is it endemic to adolescents or to institutions. Many offenders, retardates, and psychiatric patients mutilate themselves. But so do apparently normal children, adolescents, and adults in noninstitutional settings. The phenomenon can be observed at all ages from infancy to old age.

Two important studies demonstrated very clearly that self-injurious behavior can be acquired at a very early age. Shintoub and Soulairac (1961) in following three hundred normal infants from nine months to six years observed various self-injurious behaviors (unspecified) in 11-17 percent of the group at ages nine to eighteen months. Similarly, DeLissovoy (1961) reported the frequency of self-injurious behavior in a normal population to be 15.2 percent at ages nineteen to thirty-two months.

One should not make the mistake of assuming that an act of self-mutilation typically represents an isolated phenomenon, an acute episode in the life of the mutilator. Whereas some may never repeat the single act, many others, as the following examples illustrate, continue to mutilate themselves throughout their lives, often with increasing intensity and frequency. The twenty-two mutilators studied by Bach-Y-Rita (1974) averaged 93 scars per patient with a range from 3 to 150. "Most of the patients had so many scars that they had become confluent and difficult to count" (p. 108). Lovaas and Simmons (1969) noted that one patient, an eight-year-old boy, hit his head against his crib and beat his head with his fist nearly ten thousand times within a fifteen-hour "extinction phase" spread over a ten-day period. A thirty-three-year-old retarded female who was treated by Rechter and Vrablic (1974) had spent thirteen years of her life in institutions *in restraints* because of the persistence and the severity of her self-mutilatory behavior. At one point this woman split a ¾-inch thick table with her head and on another occasion dented a steel bedstead, also with her head.

Table 3–1
Incidence

Type	*Population*	*Settings*	*Incidence*	*Source*
Correctional Settings				
Cutting Ingesting/inserting Burning Constricting Hitting	Women offenders	Holloway Prison	48 in 6 months by 39 subjects $\bar{X}$ = 1.5 per week $\bar{X}$ population = 321	Cookson (1977)
Cutting Ingesting/inserting Hitting Constricting Burning	Adult male offenders	Kansas State Prison	92 incidents in 1 year by 38 inmates	Atkins (1978)
Cutting Ingesting/inserting Constricting Burning Severing Hitting	Adult male offenders	North Carolina-Ivey Bluff Maximum Security Prison	291 prisoners in 7½ years 11.2% of white inmates 1.1% of black inmates	Johnson (1973)
Various	Habitually violent patient/inmates	California Department of Corrections, Special Handling Unit	375 of a group of 22 during admission/intake	Bacy-Y-Rita (1974)
Various	Habitually violent patient/inmates	California Department of Corrections, Special Handling Unit	42% of a group of 62 in-patients	Bach-Y-Rita and Vero (1974)
Psychiatric Hospitals				
Biting	Psychiatric patients	Psychiatric Hospital	7.4% were nail biters n = 598	Ballinger (1970)
Various	Psychiatric patients	New York Psychiatric Hospital	4.29% of 2,816 patients	Phillips and Muzaffer (1961)

Hitting	Schizophrenic children (ages 5–12)	Ittleson center	10-year period 40% of population of 70	Green (1967)
Cutting	Psychiatric patients	Large Psychiatric Hospital	4.3% (121 persons) of population n = 2,816	Phillips and Muzaffer (1961)
Cutting Ingesting/inserting	Emotionally disturbed adolescents (13–16 years)	Adolescent Psychiatric Unit	11 of 25 children multiple occurrences per child	Matthews (1968)
Various	Mentally ill	Royal Dundee Liff (Psychiatric Hospital, Scotland	3% of population during 1 month n = 598	Ballinger (1971)
Various	Psychiatric patients	Chicago, Michael Reese Hospital	90 incidents between November 1958 and August 1959	Offer and Barlow (1960)
Cutting	Psychiatric patients	Chestnut Lodge Great Britain (Psychiatric Hospital)	10-year period: 1957 to 1966 32 of 413 new admissions (7.7%)	Pao (1969)
Ocular self-enucleation	Psychotics	Varied	Pre-1933 4 enucleated both eyes, 17 only one eye	Goodhart and Savitsky (1933)
			Post-1933 to 1971 9 cases reported	Carson and Lewis (1971)
Institutions for Retarded				
Various	1. Patients with Cornelia de Lange syndrome 2. Severely retarded patients	California Hospital for Severe Retardates	1. 4 out of 7 patients with syndrome self-mutilated 2. 10% of 2,000 patients	Bryson, et al. (1971)
Cutting	Febbleminded children and adolescents	School for retardates	2.1% of population	Ressman and Butterworth (1952)
Various	Mentally subnormal patients	Strathmartine Hospital, Dundee, Great Britain	15% of population in one month, n = 631	Ballinger (1971)
General Noninstitution Populations				
Hitting	Normal infants 8 months to 25 months	Private medical practice	3.6% of cases studied n = 1,168	Kravitz et al. (1960)

Table 3–1, continued
Incidence

Type	*Population*	*Settings*	*Incidence*	*Source*
General Noninstitution Populations, continued				
Biting	Normal school children	Schools	Increasing incidence of nail-biting with a peak of 45% at 12 years of age	Wechsler (1931)
Various	Normal infants	Community	Self-injurious behavior was observed in 11% to 17% of group at ages 9–18 months; 9% of group at 2 years of age; and decreased thereafter; By 5 years virtually absent n = 300	Shintoub and Soulairac (1961)
Various	Normal infants	Community	15.2% of children studied aged 19–32 months, engaged in self-injurious behavior	DeLissovoy (1961)
Biting	Factory workers and students	Community	23.1% of those studied (n = 723) were nail biters	Ballinger (1970)
Head banging	Normal infants	Community	Followed up a sample of new-borns for 20 to 30 months; 22% of males and 7% of females were head bangers	DeLissovoy (1961)
Specialized Centers				
Various	Dermatological clinic patients	Dermatology clinics in West Germany	.06%–.34% of clinic patients	Olsen (1967)
Child-care Clinics				
Cutting Hitting	Normal children 9 months to 2 years	Child-care Center	11–17% of group age 9–18 months, 9% of group age 2 years, n = 300	Shintoub and Soulairac (1961)
Hitting	Normal children	Pediatric clinic	15–20% up to 3 years	DeLissovoy (1961)
Hitting	Normal infants	2 clinics in Illinois	2.6%–3.8% of all cases	Levy and Patrick (1949)

Various	Pediatric clinical population	Pediatric clinic	15% to 20% to the age of 2½ to 3 years	Lourie (1949)
General Hospitals				
Hitting	Normal children	General hospitals	3.5% to 6.5% of usual pediatric practice	Kravitz et al. (1960)
Ingesting and various others	Hospital admissions	General Hospital, Oxford, Great Britain	Rate of 287/100,000 persons, 1972–1973	Skrimshire (1976)
Ingesting	Hospital admissions	Royal Infirmary, Edinburgh, Great Britain	Early 1960s 500–600 yearly rate	Kessel (1966)
Cutting Inhaling Various others	Patients admitted to accident and emergency department of hospitals	City of Bristol, Great Britain	805 persons in 1972 764 perons in 1973 Peak rates Males = 334/100,000 Age 25–29 Females = 645/100,000 Age 15–29	Morgan et al. (1975) Morgan, Pocock, and Pottle (1975)
Mixed				
Various	General population	All local institutions and community reporting sources, London, Ontario	730 incidents per 100,000 population per annum 522 individuals per 100,000 population per annum	Johnson et al. (1975)
Various	General population	Various cities in Great Britain, United States, Australia	125–306 incidents per 100,000 population per annum	Whitehead, Johnson and Ferrence (1973)
Various	In-patients and out-patients	General psychiatric hospitals, Mid-Sussex, Great Britain	112 incidents per 100,000 population	Jacobson and Tribe (1972)
Dental mutilation	General population	Districts in Uganda	11.9% and 16.1% in 2 separate tribes	Pindborg (1969)

Forms

Cutting

Among the most prevalent of the forms of self-mutilation are those acts in which the individual deliberately cuts his skin. His cutting may result in minor scratches, small slits, more severe gashes, or lacerations. At the extreme are those acts in which the mutilator severs an artery or a tendon. Such acts are by no means uncommon. Sometimes only circumscribed areas are cut; sometimes the mutilator lacerates a large portion of his body with a slash. The cutting may take the form of a careful delicate incision or a grandiose slashing.

Virtually every part of the body has been subjected to self-cutting, including the face, the eyelids and the genitalia. The selection of the bodily area to cut is limited only by the dexterity of the mutilator. Ironically, even the most severe cutting is reported to occur in the absence of pain. This is by no means simply because the perpetrator uses sharp instruments or mildly anesthetizes his skin by immersion in cold water. By far the majority of skin-cutting is performed with crude, dull instruments and without any attempt to desensitize the skin before it is lacerated. The depth of the incision is testimony to the characteristic ability of the mutilator to withstand what would be excruciating pain for most individuals. A recent report by Jones (1976) illustrates that the cutting behavior of self-mutilators can resemble a surgical procedure which for most people would have required total anesthesia. Jones reports the self-inflicted wound of an inmate in a correctional institution:

> [it] consisted of an opening in the abdomen perhaps three inches in diameter and with the upper circumference extending to perhaps an inch below the navel. The researcher was introduced to the prisoner who offered to expose the wound for examination. He proceeded to unfasten a wide belt, which in turn released several pieces of four inch gauze used to plug the opening. He reclined on his back, removed the final gauze, and several fluid ounces of liquid feces were ejaculated into the air, because of puncture holes in his colon. Then the feces drained back into the cavity, which the prisoner repacked with gauze. [P. 74]

As you will see, a variety of reports have been subsumed under our behavioral-descriptive classification of cutting. The choice of terms, such as cutting, scratching, lacerating, or wounding, were as likely, we discovered, to reflect the language preference of the investigator as to imply some dimension of size, length, or severity of the cut inflicted by the mutilator. Some investigators do, in fact, refer specifically to an act of self-cutting (Cookson, 1977; McKerracher, Loughane, and Watson, 1968; Money, Wolff, and Annecillo, 1972). Pao (1969) has even proposed a differentiation between self-cutting patterns which reflect more potentially serious behavior involving "a life-endangering cut" as distinct from "a superficial, delicate, carefully designed incision" (p. 9).

The term cutting, then, describes the behavioral event. Despite the awkwardness of the term in distinguishing it from similar behaviors such as abrading, severing parts of the body, or inserting objects under the skin, it appears to be useful in integrating an otherwise disparate set of behaviors. For example, instances of cutting of the face have included direct facial incisions (Cox and Klinge, 1976; Novotny, 1972; Podvoll, 1969; Roback et al., 1972; Rosenthal et al., 1972); scratching of the facial areas (Corte, Wolff, and Locke, 1971; Crabtree, 1967; Rosenthal et al., 1972); pricking of the face (Hawkins, Jones, and Tibbetts, 1956); and cutting of the eyelid (Atkins, 1978). Mutilators have also cut or slashed their necks (Atkins, 1978; Novotny, 1972; Rosenthal et al., 1972) and upper back and shoulders (Ragain and Anson, 1976).

Miller and Bashkin, (1975) discuss a client who had a penchant for arm cutting:

> At the first interview he wore a short-sleeved shirt and conspicuously displayed his injuries. He seemed proud of them, not embarassed and conveyed the impression that he saw them to be, as it were, medals of honor received in the line of duty. [P. 640]

The arm is a site frequently selected by the mutilator. The female adolescent offenders at Grandview exhibited a preference for carving their arms, as do adolescents in psychiatric units (Matthews, 1968).

There are a number of conjectural reasons for this preference. The arm is easily accessible and can be readily observed during the act of cutting. It does not require any great dexterity to inflict a wound in this area. It is also a highly visible location, yet it has the distinct advantage of selective exposure through an appropriate choice of clothing. Some of our girls with carving scars on their arms would deliberately adopt a style of dress which would accentuate the shock value of their cuts, such as short-sleeved or tank-top shirts. Some would even choose the color of their clothes in order to provide a bold contrast with their scars. Others preferred to cover the scarred areas with entirely appropriate clothing such as long-sleeved sweaters. The unsuspecting visitor would then be shocked when an otherwise nicely attired, attractive teenage girl would suddenly roll up her sleeves to expose her scarred arms. It had, more often that we care to remember, the desired effect. It also accomplished an important ancillary purpose. It embarassed their keepers. As we noted earlier, the staff felt compelled to hide the evidence of carving whenever the girls met the public or the public met the girls. If a carver could not be prevented from such contacts, she would be dressed in a manner designed to minimize the impact of her scars. As you can readily imagine, with our enterprising young ladies, such efforts, albeit well intentioned, were futile.

Bach-Y-Rita (1974) and Bach-Y-Rita and Veno (1974), in a comprehensive study of habitually violent offenders in the California penal system, have also drawn attention to the prevalence of arm slashing. Their observations have received considerable support in studies conducted in a wide variety of settings and among diverse populations (Ball et al., 1975; Cox and Klinge, 1976; Crabtree, 1967; Kafka, 1969; Novotny, 1972; Offer and Barlow, 1960; Panton, 1962; Rosenthal et al., 1972; Siomopoulous, 1974).

Scratching (Asch, 1971), cutting and slashing (Nelson and Grunebaum, 1971) of the wrist area is more widely known as a self-inflicted injury. It is clearly recognized as a frequent choice in suicide attempts or gestures (Greer and Lee, 1967; Kessel, 1966; Simpson, 1973; Virkkunen, 1976) and has even led some investigators to propose a wrist-cutting syndrome (Pao, 1969; Rosenthal et al., 1972). Ryback (1971) reports a case of a thirty-two-year-old truck driver who slashed his wrists while in an alcohol-induced amnesic state. He could only remember that he had been drinking at the bar and then found himself:

> . . . standing in his apartment with the telephone in his hand saying "there's blood on the damned phone . . ." He did not know to whom he was talking nor did he remember driving to his apartment or cutting his wrists with a razor blade. [P. 533]

Cutting behavior has also localized on the hand and parts of the hand Matthews, 1968; Rosenthal et al., 1972). There are many documented instances of thumb cutting (Atkins, 1978), finger cutting (Offer and Barlow, 1960; Tate, 1972) and cutting of the thumb tendon (Atkins, 1978). Goldfarb (1958) describes a patient:

> Benny came to me with scissors and asked me to cut. He was cutting the palm of his left hand till he had produced a bleeding gash. He showed no reaction of pain, even when the gash was cleaned. [P. 779]

Clinical examples of repeated self-cutting of the breast and chest area have been reported by Simpson (1973) and Siomopoulos (1974). Miller and Bashkin (1974) describe a twenty-nine-year-old male patient:

> Twenty-two months were marked by severe and incessant self-mutilations. During this period the patient inflicted hundreds of wounds on his arms, legs, chest and abdomen. On occasion, the abdominal lacerations penetrated the peritoneum. The wounds on his chest exposed ribs. [P. 640]

Similar reports of chest cutting (Atkins, 1978; Panton, 1962) and stabbing (Greer and Lee, 1967) would seem to indicate that this form of self-mutilation is not uncommon. One case of navel cutting was located where: "one patient from age eight had pricked her navel with a pin until blood appeared" (Novotny, 1972, p. 107). In addition there have been numerous instances which involve cutting in the area of the abdomen (Atkins, 1978; Gardner and Gardner, 1975; Miller and Bashkin, 1974; Novotny, 1972; Panton, 1962; Siomopoulos, 1974), thighs (Roback et al., 1972), and various parts of the legs (Gardner and Gardner, 1975; Kafka, 1969; Miller and Bashkin, 1974; Novotny, 1972).

Several investigators have reported instances of self-cutting of the vaginal area (for example, Simpson, 1973). Feet have been scratched and cut (Claghorn and Beto, 1967), Achilles tendons lacerated (Atkins, 1978; Clanon, 1965), and the soles of the foot have suffered effects of walking on glass (Shah and Rohter, 1978). No part of the body is immune to the efforts of a determined mutilator.

A mutilator intent on inflicting cuts on his body is rarely deterred by the lack of an instrument to perform the task. Scratching with a fingernail will suffice. Allen and Harris (1966) present the case of a child who "for almost a year, had been scratching until she bled. The scratching behavior had resulted in large sores and scabs on her forehead, nose, cheeks, chin and one arm and leg" (p. 80). Azrin et al. (1975), Crabtree (1967), and Shodell and Reiter (1968) have documented similar cases.

Medical treatment for their wounds may not deter the mutilator. He may simply remove the sutures to ensure further damage (Atkins, 1978; Rosenthal et al., 1972; Simpson, 1973). Finally, many reports of cutting do not specify a target area and, as macabre as it may seem, simply describe the patients as being "cut everywhere" (Jacobson and Tribe, 1972; Johnson et al., 1975; Morgan, Pocock, and Pottle, 1975; and Morgan et al., 1975).

Biting

As noted, the lack of an instrument for cutting presents no serious obstacle to the determined mutilator. Most have built-in cutting instruments: their teeth. What can chew and tear food can chew and tear flesh just as efficiently. In fact, Tate (1972) describes the use of dental surgery as a controlling strategy for self-mutilators: their teeth were extracted!

Most readers will, of course, be familiar with one form of self-biting: nail biting. This behavior illustrates very clearly the range of severity of self-mutilatory behavior. Some nail biting represents a rather crude form of self-grooming in which the individual controls the length of his nails with his teeth rather than with nail clippers or scissors. At the other extreme are those instances in which the nails are bitten to such an extent that little of the nail itself is left, the fingers are bitten to the cuticles, and the nail bed skin is chewed (Money, Wolff, and Annecillo, 1972).

Some of the reports of self-biting were so repugnant or repulsive to our research staff that they immediately passed them to us to handle. In spite of our experience with self-mutilatory behavior, even we had difficulty in reading the material. Particularly was this the case when accompanying the report were photographs of patients who had bitten off chunks of skin or had literally devoured their fingers or tongues. For instance, Slawson and Davidson (1964) describe a young woman who had repeatedly bitten her own tongue. She had to use her fingers to pry open her jaw when requested to display her tongue. It was macerated, its edges were jagged, and the tip had been bitten off.

> . . . her speech was garbled and halting. Unable to eat or drink . . . she was malnourished and dehydrated. When a bite occurred, as they did two or three times each hour, she would cry out in excruciating pain, protrude her tongue, and expose chunks of freshly lacerated bleeding tissue." [P. 581]

Individuals have chewed their nails, their hands, their lips, their shoulders, their tongues, and the inner parts of their mouths. The only limitation to the variety of self-mutilation through biting is the ability of the body to contort.

The occurrence of self-biting among mentally retarded patients has been reported by many investigators (for example, Azrin et al., 1975; Lovaas and Simmons, 1969). Self-biting is often reported in schizophrenic children (for example, Green, 1968; Lovaas and Simmons, 1969; Shodell and Reiter, 1968). Self-biting behaviors have also been observed in very young children. Duker (1975), for example, has reported the case of self-biting in a retarded male at age one and a half. However, such behavior is not limited to children. Cautela and Baron (1973) have described a twenty-year-old male college student who bit his tongue on a daily basis over a six-month period. This schizophrenic patient had been placed in restraints to prevent other self-damaging behavior and soon began biting his lips and tongue to the point where "he had completely bitten off some lower lip tissue and a considerable portion of the upper lip. Resultant scar-tissue formation had reduced the size of his mouth opening to one-half" (p. 127).

Destructive lip biting is always found in the Lesh-Nyhan syndrome (Bryson et al., 1971). Examples of self-biting have been reported by Cooper and Fowlie (1973) and by Sandow (1975).

Betts's (1964) term *autocannibalism* is not a mere metaphor.

Abrading

Perhaps the most common intervention technique employed in attempts to control or prevent self-mutilation is security. Mutilators have been isolated, stripped, denied access to potential instruments, locked in rooms, drugged, tied to beds, dressed in restrictive clothing (such as mitts, helmets, straight jackets, body casts) and kept under immediate personal surveillance. Such security techniques are often impressively ineffective in deterring the self-mutilator. There are always objects that the mutilator can rub his body against with abrasive effect. Severe abrasions can be readily engendered by brisk or prolonged rubbing of the body against furniture, floors, walls, or even against one's own body. Constant irritation of the skin by licking, sucking, rubbing, or gouging can readily lead to open wounds and sores. Many a parent can attest to thumb-sucking children who have made both their thumbs and their lips raw by prolonged or intense sucking. Many a nurse has had a patient whose wound would not heal because the patient aggravated it by rubbing (Kafka, 1971). Each of us has also probably experienced sores which we have created by injudiciously rubbing or scratching a minor skin irritation. These are apparently normal experiences which we all share. Dermatologists, gynecologists, plastic surgeons, and others have frequently encountered patients who have done remarkable damage to themselves by deliberately abrading various parts of their body.

Eye irritation in the absence of any apparent organic cause is frequently observed. Such irritation can be caused by the patient deliberately and persistently rubbing his eyes (Cautela and Baron, 1973).

A case of vaginal abrading is reported by Money, Wolff, and Annecillo, (1972). In this case, a female child participated in such behavior at the age of five. The behavior involved "excessive masturbation" to the point where the subject's vaginal infection resulted in painful urination. Rosenthal et al., (1972) have described twenty-three female psychiatric in-patients (mean age: twenty-two years) who abraded themselves by "scratching, gouging, or rubbing glass fragments into their faces" (p. 1364).

Bryson et al., (1971) noted in their study of the Cornelia de Lange syndrome a patient who rubbed her cheek with the back of her hands for hours at a time. The effect was "reddening, excoriation, abrasion, bleeding, and secondary infection. She maintained this habit for years . . . . all treatments failed to clear the dermatitis because her rubbing was persistent." [p. 321]

Severing

Many self-mutilating acts lead to bodily damage which is permanent and unalterable. Clearly this is the case with self-mutilation in which fingers, toes, ears, tongues, or genitals are severed, as it is in self-mutilation involving disembowling or eye enucleation. Such acts are particularly abhorrent and conjure up notions of psychopathology. However, before we automatically assume that such acts are an affront to normality or sanity we should recall some of the doctrines for appeasement of sin which are proclaimed in the Bible. For example, the recommended treatments for adultery (which according to the New Testament merely includes looking at a woman "to lust after her") are: self-enucleation of the eye(s) and self-amputation of hands and feet.

Some self-mutilators take biblical exhortations literally. Voluntary castration was prevalent as a means of obtaining the lucrative and powerful position as a eunuch in the imperial court. In Russia in the nineteenth century castration was popular among early Christian sects. In the sixteenth and seventeenth centuries young boys often sought castration in order to preserve their soprano voices. Breast removal, often through self-surgery, is well known in Amazon women. (Amazon literally means "without breasts)".

Often an act of severing represents a single and isolated mutilatory response in an individual without a history of self-mutilation. However, in some exceptional cases the severing is not an impulsive act but one in a series of acts in which the individual has deliberately and systematically severed various parts of his body. One of our respondents referred to such a case, not altogether facetiously, as the "case of the rapidly diminishing client."

Blacker and Wong (1963) describe four severe cases of autocastration in borderline or psychotic patients. One case slashed his left testicle, then cut his penis with a butcher knife. Next he cut his scrotum and removed the remaining testicle. In a coup de grace "he drove to a wooded area, tied a string about his penis until it became numb, and then amputated it close to his body" (p. 171). A second patient "placed his penis on a wood block and chopped at the base with a hatchet. He stopped when he saw blood, more out of fear than pain, and staggered off to bed still bleeding. His former wife telephoned that evening, sensed that something was wrong, and called the police who took him to a general hospital where he was given three units of blood" (p. 172). A third case "amputated his penis with a razor" and still another case is described as follows: "on hearing both a male and a female voice planning to possess his genitalia for their own purposes, he experienced a 'burning sensation' in his penis and became anxious. Then, panic-stricken, he ligated it with string and proceeded to incise his scrotum to free himself of the 'spirits' ' influence. Still not satisfied he had begun to amputate his penis with a razor when he was discovered by his sister" (p. 173). Accounts of incidents of autocastration have also been provided by Helzel (1978), Schott (1973), and Yaroshevsky (1975).

Less dramatic but also permanently damaging acts include severing of nails (Lovaas and Simmons, 1969), toes (Yaroshevsky, 1975; Johnson, 1975), and fingers (Lovaas and Simmons, 1969; Yaroshevsky, 1975). The severing of the ear by the artist van Gogh is well known. (Lubin, 1961). Other cases have been reported (Critchley, 1934).

We have described the case of the hysterical twenty-nine-year-old woman who bit off the tip of her tongue (Slawson and Davidson, 1964). Michael and Beck (1973) also report a case of a thirty-three-year-old male who cut out the anterior two-thirds of his tongue with razor blades. Such self-severing has also been observed in infancy. Neil (1958) describes a patient who when left alone in his cot began self-biting, resulting in "almost complete destruction of the tip of the tongue, leaving a raw, irregular, granulated surface." The patient was thirteen months old. Completing the anatomical inventory are those nonsuicidal cases of partial disembowling which have been reported (for example, Yaroshevsky, 1975).

The classification of one variety of self-mutilatory behavior, hair pulling, was problematic (Corte, Wolff, and Locke; Cox and Klinge, 1976; Goldfarb, 1958). We decided to view hair pulling as a type of severing since it does entail removal of bodily parts, but in so doing we clearly recognize the shortcomings of the behavioral classification schema we have adopted.

Inserting

A startling array of objects, including needles, pins, nails, paper clips, and glass, have been inserted under the skin by self-mutilators. Sometimes the objects are inserted in such a way that they create what to the mutilator's perception is a bodily decoration. For example, at an institution for retarded adolescent girls, many patients created what appeared to be belts by inserting pins under the skin around their midriffs. The belt was completed by a number of larger pins placed at right angles to each other to form a buckle (Cormack, 1968). A more widely recognized self-mutilatory behavior is that performed by many punk rock advocates who, among other things, insert safety pins in their cheeks. Similar bodily decoration is common among primitive tribes who adorn their bodies, particularly their faces, with animal bones inserted under the skin.

Inserting, unlike many other forms of self-mutilation, is often done cautiously and slowly rather than impulsively. It often reflects care and precision. Moreover, these mutilators frequently plan their act, even plot it well in advance as, for example, when they steal and hide objects which they wish to implant. The care that is required is well reflected in the case of a mutilator who literally sewed buttons on his body (Yaroshevsky, 1975). There are, of course, many cases where the mutilator inserts an object in his body in an impulsive manner in apparent exception to the more typical inserter whose self-mutilation is both stylistic (in his view) and ritualistic.

An impressive array of objects have been inserted in bodily orifices—the vagina, the navel, and the anus. This is by no means an uncommon behavior, and in the vast majority of instances it is not self-mutilatory either by intention or by consequence. What may merely be playful or exploratory behavior on the part of a child or self-stimulatory behavior in an older person may be self-mutilatory if there is some deliberate attempt to injure oneself. They should be differentiated from cases in which the individual has injured himself accidentally by the injudicious insertion of potentially harmful objects. The difference between a self-harming act committed by an individual with limited understanding of anatomy, limited common sense, poor judgment, poor motor skills, or simple bad luck and a similar act perpetrated by an individual who deliberately intends to injure himself highlights the difficulty in attempting to classify or diagnose self-injurious behavior. Two different labels (self-mutilation and accidental injury) may be applied to the same response.

Regardless of the labeling or definitional problems, there are many reports of individuals who have very deliberately injured themselves by inserting obviously dangerous objects in their bodily orifices. For example, Simpson (1973) described Mary D., a patient who on various occasions had introduced a spring, a knitting needle, a sewing needle, hat pins, and a kitchen knife into her vagina. She "admitted to planning most incidents carefully, enjoying the anticipation of the event" (p. 809).

Long needles and steel bristles have been inserted into limbs (Hawkins, Jones, and Tibbetts, 1956); glass fragments have been rubbed permanently into the face (Rosenthal et al., 1972); pins have been inserted into the forearms or face (Matthews, 1968); nails and paper clips have been inserted into the abdomen (Johnson, 1973); and, in some instances, objects have been deliberately inserted in the urethra (Johnson, 1973). Nails have even been inserted in the cheeks in an apparent reenactment of crucifixion. (Shah and Rohter, 1978).

Burning

Often the self-mutilator is sufficiently in control of his injurious behavior that he can guarantee his safety and ensure that the resultant damage is in keeping with his intent. He merely stops when he has "had enough." However, in a great many instances the mutilator ends up much more seriously damaged than he intended (either through naivete or accident). Such is the case, for instance, when the act involves swallowing sharp objects such as glass. Once initiated, the damaging action cannot be voluntarily and easily controlled or terminated. Dramatic examples of the irreversibility of a self-mutilating act are found in cases of self-burning where the mutilator, intent on burning only part of his body, starts an action that leads to his burning a major part of his body surface. For example, he spills the flammable fluid over onto other parts of his body and his clothes ignite. Some cases of total immolation may have been inadvertent exaggerations of more minor intentional self-mutilatory behavior reflecting the individual's inability to stop an action he initiated—a relatively insignificant act gets out of control. The conservative burner often walks a thin line between self-injury and self-destruction.

Total self-immolation is an extreme and sensational form of self-burning. More common is minor burning of small portions of the skin typically carried out with cigarettes or matches. Unlike some forms of self-mutilation which require prolonged effort or preparation, burning can be initiated impulsively and completed quickly. Moreover, the effect is immediately apparent. Interestingly, many self-burners report that more pain ensues from the treatment of the resulting burns than was experienced in the self-mutilating act itself.

Self-burners often have a considerable flair for the dramatic, as when they turn themselves into a ball of fire or when, in a display of machismo, they thrust their hands into open flames. Gross disfigurement often results from such behavior. Apparently the most popular method of self-burning is to use lighted cigarettes (Asch, 1971; Claghorn and Beto, 1967; Green, 1968, Rosenthal et al., 1972). Other methods include sitting on hot radiators (Hawkins, et al., 1956), ingesting boiling hot soup (Money, et al., 1972), and pouring caustic potash in superficial lacerations of the arms and legs (Panton, 1962). Burns have also been induced by the application to the skin of nitric acid (Hawkins, Jones, and Tibbetts, 1956). One correctional inmate was reported to have burned himself by wrapping toilet paper around his wrist and lighting it (Johnson, 1973). Hot metals have also been deliberately applied to the skin (Johnson, 1973; Rosenthal et al., 1972), and individuals have walked on hot coals (Shah and Rohter, 1978). A simple method involves setting one's clothes on fire (Battle and Marshall, 1952; Bostic, 1973; Claghorn and Beto, 1967). Self-induced electric shocks can also result in burns (Jacobson and Tribe, 1972). As is the case in most forms of self-mutilation, no part of his body is safe from the attack of the self-burner. The hands, the arms, the thighs, the feet, the stomach, and even the face have been targets (Cox and Klinge, 1976; Roback et al., 1972).

Ingesting or Inhaling

The hackles of the nutritionist would likely be raised by the diet of some self-mutilators. Mutilators have managed to swallow an incredible array of objects which most of us would prefer to associate with locations far removed from our stomachs. The materials range from pins and needles to faucet handles.

The effects of swallowing such indigestible objects can be lethal, and often are. Fatal or not, the intestinal damage that can be wrought by the ingestion of glass, caustic substances, and other objects distinctly foreign to the normal stomach or bowel is horrifying. A wide variety of drugs have been included in some self-mutilator's self-prescribed, self-abusive diet: tranquilizers (Bean, 1974); excessive amounts of cough medicine (Offer and Barlow, 1960); and innumerable pills (Atkins, 1978; Bancroft et al., 1975; Cookson, 1977; Friedman et al., 1972; Green, 1967; Jacobson, and Tribe, 1972; Johnson et al., 1975; Kafka, 1969; Kessel, 1966; Matthews, 1968; Money, Wolff, and Annecillo, 1972; Morgan, Pocock, and Pottle, 1975; Morgan et al., 1975).

The deliberately excessive ingestion of aspirins, taken by themselves or in combination with alcohol (Simpson, 1973), is commonplace in the observations of most physicians. Included in such preferences have been solvents, acids, and weed killers (Bean, 1974), needles (Crabtree, 1967), cyanide (Friedman et al., 1972), thyroid extract and laxatives (Hawkins, Jones, and Tibbetts, 1956), and stones (Money, Wolff, and Annecillo, 1972). The menu for some self-mutilators has included mercury extracted from the base of a thermometer (Johnson, 1973), light bulbs (Shah and Rohter, 1978), feces and urine (Atkins, 1978), a spring (Simpson, 1973), drawing pins (Matthews, 1968), hair (Green, 1968), screws and nails (Shah and Rohter, 1978), and faucet handles (Johnson, 1973).

Yaroshevsky (1975), a Canadian doctor who was imprisoned in the U.S.S.R. from 1958 to 1961, discovered, while serving as the prison surgeon, a bewildering variety of objects (glass, razor blades, nails, spoons, thermometers, and wire) had been swallowed with a methodical technique:

> The prisoner inserts the nail (or other similar objects, such as a spoon or knife) into his throat with its blunt end down. He then places his finger on the other end, quickly presses down on the point and makes a swallowing movement. [P. 445]

Severe internal damage can also be occasioned by the mutilator who deliberately inhales various gases (Alderson, 1974; Bean, 1974; Green, 1967; Jacobson and Tribe, 1972; Jarvis et al., 1976; Johnson et al., 1975; Morgan, Pocock, and Pottle, 1975; Morgan et al., 1975).

Hitting

One of the most studied self-mutilatory behaviors is head banging. Head banging is also very familiar to the layperson. Most people have known of children who engage in banging of their heads against the headboards of beds or who, while sitting, rock themselves continuously against the back of chairs. Such behavior is only too common in institutions for retarded and autistic children. We classify such behavior as self-mutilatory rather than merely self-stimulatory to acknowledge the fact that such behavior can and too frequently does lead to serious physical damage during contusions, hematomas, and loosening of retinas. At the same time it should be recognized that this behavior in milder or less frequent form is highly prevalent in healthy children. Self-mutilatory behavior does not necessarily differ qualitatively from other behaviors.

There are many reasons why investigators have focused so much attention on head banging. One reason is that unlike many other forms of self-mutilation, it is highly public and occurs with such frequency that it lends itself readily to research. Social scientists, particularly behaviorists, are attracted to things they can count and translate into graphs and tables. They also seem to be motivated to investigate behaviors which are annoying. Head banging, because of its repetitive nature and its resistance to treatment, can be especially annoying, as parents and institutional attendants know only too well. Short of physically immobilizing the head banger, there is little the distressed adults feel they can do to stop the thumping of the head banger, and it often continues uninterruptedly hour after hour throughout the night. It is not merely annoying; it is frightening. It stimulates horrendous fantasies in peoples' minds, including notions that the head banger is somehow possessed. Those who are exposed to the incessant clamor often assume, not always incorrectly, that the child may be injuring his brain.

From our point of view, head banging is only one of a wide spectrum of self-mutilations which are subsumed under our category of hitting. Such acts can occur in one or more of three possible ways:

1. Acts in which the mutilator hits his body against an object (for example, head banging, jumping from high places).
2. Objects are used to hit the body (for example, poking the eye with sticks, deliberately slamming doors on fingers).
3. Parts of the body are hit by other parts of the body (for example, head and face slapping, self-kicking, or pounding the head with one's hands).

Such behaviors have been widely studied because of their frequency and because the damaging effect of such behavior is often not as readily apparent, severe, or as repugnant as is the case with lacerations or amputations. It may also be that such behaviors attract research interest because of their similarity to more socially appropriate behavior. All of us can recall slapping ourselves or kicking the furniture or, figuratively, banging our heads against the wall in mock or actual exasperation, frustration, or anger. Most of us accept without thought the players in hockey or football who hurl their bodies into or in front of their opponents, or karate enthusiasts who spend hours practicing chopping their hands against bricks or boards, or soccer players who with their unprotected heads intercept balls traveling at high velocity. The distinction between these acts and self-mutilatory acts is often blurred, except in terms of frequency, severity, or consequence.

Many individuals have sustained considerable facial damage by hitting themselves (Tate, 1972), punching themselves (Azrin et al., 1975; Merbaum, 1973), beating themselves (Claghorn and Beto, 1967; Corte, Wolff, and Locke, 1971), and slapping themselves (Azrin et al., 1975; Corte, Wolff, and Locke, 1971; Green, 1967; Lucero et al., 1976; Martin and Treffry, 1970; Romanczyk and Goren, 1975). It is not only their hands that they use:

> Her behavior over the years had come to consist mainly of compulsive hitting of her face hard enough with her fists to cause a loud cracking sound and open bleeding wounds. Her hands have been restrained . . . but she has since managed to strike herself with her knees. [Bryson et al., 1971, p. 320].

Self-mutilation by way of head hitting was reported in the case of a 49,XXXXY chromosonal constitution by Korten et al., (1975). Head slapping has been described in case reports of psychotic children (for example, Saposnek and Watson, 1974), schizophrenic adults (for example, Tanner and Zeiler, 1975), and retarded children (for example, Azrin et al., 1975; Peterson and Peterson, 1968).

The intensity that characterizes some of this behavior is dramatically portrayed in the following reports:

> From the onset he is reported to have struck his head with considerable intensity—on two separate occasions he shattered windshields and has produced dents in the interior walls of his house. [Harris and Raik 1976, p. 236]

> In addition to hitting and scratching himself . . . . Release of his legs immediately occasioned head banging with the knees. Release of his hands similarly resulted in face slapping, head knocking, or head banging with any object . . . . in various contexts—while singing, smiling, laughing, watching television, when crying alone, and with others present. [Romanczyk and Goren, 1975, p. 731]

Head banging is not only confined to the very young: Collins (1964) has observed cases of head banging in adults.

Head banging is often found in combination with other self-mutilatory behavior, for example, self-induced seizures (Gardner, 1965), torsion spasms (Duker, 1975), and body hurling (Green, 1968).

The literature on head banging is voluminous (for example, Azrin et al., 1975; Cox and Klinge, 1976; Duker, 1975; Fielding and Cole, 1971; Green, 1968; Harris and Raik, 1976; Johnson, 1973; Lovaas and Simmons, 1969; Martin and Treffry, 1970; Money, Wolff, and Annecillo, 1972; Morrison, 1972; Muttar et al., 1975; Peterson and Peterson, 1968; Ragain and Anson, 1976; Romanczyk and Goren, 1975; Ross, Meichenbaum, Humphreys, 1971; Sandow, 1975; Shodell and Reiter, 1968; Singh, 1976; Tate, 1972).

Ear punching has been reported by Azrin et al. (1975), Lovaas and Simmons (1969), and Lucero et al. (1976). Eye poking can have particularly unpleasant results, as is evident in this case history of a young schizophrenic:

> He was poking and/or biting almost daily. He had completely lost the sight of one eye and inflammation of the other eye prevented a definite assessment of his status. [Cautela and Baron, 1973, p. 126-127]

Eye banging was investigated by Stinnett and Hollender (1970) who report the case of a young man who had the compulsion to hit his eyes:

He hit them with such force and frequency that he produced bilateral retinal detachments and traumatic cataracts resulting in a complete loss of vision in one eye and a sixty percent loss in the other. [P. 371]

Instances of arm banging occur in case studies by Atkins (1978) and Lovaas and Simmons (1969). Self-mutilation may also occur by way of hand pounding (Green, 1968), hitting the hand against teeth (Jones, Simmons, and Frankel, 1974; Peterson and Peterson, 1968), jabbing (Jones, Simmons, and Frankel, 1974), and knuckle banging (Offer and Barlow, 1960).

One young schizophrenic child repeatedly stuck her fingers in doors:

Alice caught her finger in the door. The tip was cut and the finger was swollen and blue. She did not cry at the time of the accident, nor when the wound was dressed. Later, she was observed smilingly looking at the finger with no report of pain. [Goldfarb, 1958, p. 778]

Common in the literature are reports of individuals damaging their legs by kicking solid objects or damaging other parts of their bodies by self-kicking (Green, 1967; Peterson and Peterson, 1968).

Tate (1972) describes the following case:

When her leg was released from restraints, Suzie kicked herself and any hard object in reach. She kicked the side of the bed, her other leg and foot, and her crotch. During a 7 hour 33 minutes observation period . . . . she kicked 5,866 times. [P. 74]

The patient's kicking was severe, producing wounds in spite of four inch thick protective foam padding on the limbs. Free from restraint she would use her knees to hit her head with sufficient force to engender hematomas.

Many individuals cause damage to themselves by deliberately falling (Johnson, 1973; Money, Wolff, and Annecillo, 1972; Sandow, 1975), or by failing to protect themselves when falling (Money, Wolff, and Annecillo, 1972), or by deliberately jumping under circumstances which are almost guaranteed to result in injury but not death (for example, Novotny, 1972).

Constricting

Frequently in the literature on suicide one finds reference to self-destruction by means of suffocation, drowning, or hanging. Seldom in discussions of self-mutilation do investigators refer to nonfatal instances of such behavior. Typically, nonfatal occurrences are viewed as attempted but unsuccessful suicide in spite of the fact that some individuals often commit such acts without the slightest intention of dying or even of making people think they were intending to die.

Scattered along throughout the literature are reports of individuals who have deliberately injured themselves by acts which involve constricting the flow of blood to parts of their body, or constricting their air passages in various ways. The effects of such behaviors are often relatively minor, but they can engender rather serious long-term effects and can inadverdently or accidentally lead to death.

Hawkins, Jones, and Tibbetts (1956) report the case of a patient who suffered from numbness, stiffness, and cyanosis in her arms, produced by tying bands around her upper arms. Other methods of constricting include winding a rubber band around the thumb to make it fall off (Matthews, 1968), mouth sewing (Yaroshevsky, 1975), and pinching the skin to cut off the flow of blood (Jones, Simmons, and Frankel, 1974).

A grim yet inventive instance of self-inflicted frostbite, which has the effect of constricting the flow of blood, is chronicled by Yaroshevsky (1975):

> Another young prisoner.... urinated on his feet, then put them through a broken window during January when the temperature fell below freezing and was badly frostbitten. He was treated in hospital for about nine months and suffered permanent damage. [P. 445]

Self-injury by way of strangulation (Cookson, 1977; Jacobson and Tribe, 1972), water immersion (Morgan, Pocock, and Pottle, 1975; Morgan et al., 1975; Johnson et al., 1975; Jacobson and Tribe, 1972), and hanging (Atkins, 1978; Johnson et al., 1975) is certainly not unusual. However, decidedly more uncommon are instances wherein individuals have injured themselves by deliberately restricting their oxygen supply in order to increase sexual arousal. Edmondson described the following case of a fourteen-and-a-half-year-old boy:

> He had been surprised by his mother who found him lying on his back clearly in the process of masturbating. He had a rope passing around the end of his bed and then round his neck under his chin, and he was blue in the face. [Edmondson, 1972, p. 437]

Jayewardene (1978) has pointed out that a verdict of intentional suicide has been reached in cases where individuals in the process of engendering anoxia in order to heighten sexual stimulation at the point of orgasm lost control and accidentally hung themselves.

No doubt this chapter on the variety of forms of self-mutilation could be continued ad infinitum (if not ad nauseum). As we noted earlier, it has not been our intention to be exhaustive in listing or describing the vagaries of self-mutilating behavior. Rather, our goal has been to help the reader view the carving behavior of our adolescent girls within a broader perspective.

Before concluding this chapter we would like to debunk a myth. The occurrence of carving and other self-mutilatory behavior among the girls at Grandview was often used by the critics of training schools to substantiate their views that such institutions should be abolished because, they asserted, it is the training school environment that is solely responsible for engendering self-mutilatory behavior. We admit to having shared that view occasionally. We do not wish to deny the fact that the training school environment contributes to the occurrence of self-mutilation. However, this chapter documents the fact that self-mutilation is not an isolated phenomenon. Self-mutilation is much more prevalent than we might suspect; it takes myriad forms and occurs in diverse settings and among heterogeneous populations. The cases we have described clearly demonstrate the shortsightedness of the view that self-mutilatory behavior is strictly a training school phenomenon. Such simple explanations do not do justice to the complexity of the phenomenon. Many of the other forms of self-mutilation had been demonstrated by the Grandview girls long before they arrived at our doors. Perhaps carving represents a situationally sanctioned, topographically distinct form of self-mutilation: the training school variety of self-mutilatory behavior.

By reviewing the literature on self-mutilation we may not have made the task of explaining our adolescents' carving any easier. We are now faced with the problem of trying to find an explanation for the carving at Grandview which will allow us to understand similar behavior in other populations in other settings. It is unlikely that an explanation that is situationally specific will be of much value. On the other hand, attempting to find more inclusive explanations for such a heterogeneity of behaviors is a formidable task. Indeed we must seriously question whether such topographically distinct behaviors really share any common motivational base.

4 Explanations of Self-Mutilation

The Plogglies

The discovery of plogglies was first reported by the eminent linguist Wendel Johnson (1946) in his book *People in Quandries*, in which he described to the scientific community the solution to two mysteries. The mysteries had been a source of considerable social irritation and had for many years perplexed rational men who had devoted their lives to their study.

> The mysteries were that whenever anyone wanted to find a lead pencil he couldn't, and whenever anyone wanted to sharpen a lead pencil the sharpener was sure to be filled with pencil shavings. [P. 76]

In response to public pressure the government appointed a committee of distinguished philosophers to seek an explanation of the mysteries.

Following months of detailed investigation of all the circumstances surrounding the mystery, and countless interviews with the people who had personally been affected by the vexing problem, the committee was finally able to solve the mystery. Their explanation, like many great breakthroughs, was both simple and brilliant:

> Beneath the ground, so the theory went, live a great number of little people. They are called plogglies. At night, explained the philosophers, when people are asleep, the plogglies come into their houses. They scurry around and gather up all the lead pencils, and then they scamper over to the pencil sharpener and grind them all up. And then they go back into the ground. [P. 76]

As Johnson points out, this was a remarkable theory which could explain both mysteries. The public was relieved that the mysteries had been solved, and their agitation of the government quickly subsided. Now that they understood the cause of the problem they could live with it.

The discovery of plogglies also helped the government to explain the failure of their attempts to protect the public's pencils. It was because "Plogglies are like that," "It is the plogglies' will," "You can expect that with plogglies," and "What can you do with plogglies?"

The discovery of plogglies proved to be a thoroughly satisfactory explanation—at least for those who believed in plogglies. The only trouble with the explanation is that there are no plogglies.

Plogglies in scientific parlance are hypothetical constructs. They are imaginary; fantasies that the scientist invents in order to help him to make sense out of what he observes. They can be very useful in the development of knowledge, since, for example, they make it possible for us to synthesize a mass of information which we might not otherwise be able to comprehend.

Hypothetical constructs are in fact just what the name implies–hypothetical; they may or may not exist. Whether or not plogglies actually exist or are entirely imaginary is rather immaterial. What is important is whether entertaining them as explanatory concepts leads us to develop useful ideas for controlling or predicting the phenomenon we are studying. If it helped us to find a successful remedy for self-mutilation, we would be willing to accept any explanation of self-mutilation, no matter how far-fetched.

In his chapter we will discuss the explanations that have been offered to account for the mystery as to why people actually choose to mutilate themselves. In doing so we will introduce you to a large number of ploggly-like notions which investigators have invented in an attempt to understand the rather bizarre behavior of their self-mutilating patients. Some of the constructs may seem as incredible as Wendell Johnson's plogglies, and perhaps, we should apologize for including them. However, they are frankly delightful, often ingenious, and perhaps even useful in the absence of any rival plausible hypotheses.

As you will see, some plogglies are better than others. They take many forms: commentaries, annotations, hypotheses, models, speculations, and conjectures. A few are as bizarre as some of the behaviors they seek to explain. There are as many plogglies as positors. Each has his favorite, and, we surmise, all are well intentioned. We found ourselves entertained, often persuaded, and occasionally amused by the arguments that were used to support them.

Although ploggly positors represent a wide variety of disciplines, we will not attempt to separate them here; there is nothing to be gained by doing so. Our attempts to classify the explanations were as frustrating as our attempts to treat self-mutilation.

Ritual and Symbolism

Some of the self-mutilating acts of the girls at Grandview occurred in a context of ritual, such as an initiation rite. Initiations were couched in elaborate ceremony with dramatic overtones designed to give them an aura of importance. The skilled choreography of people and events necessary to the performance of such rituals were a source of continuous astonishment to our staff. The seriousness with which the novitiate would await induction into one of these groups was ample testimony to the importance the girls attached to this peer group rite. Some ceremonies involved a group of girls sitting around in a circle, murmuring appropriate chants, followed by some prescribed pattern of behavior leading up to the final and major act of initiation—an episode of self-cutting by each member of the group. Sometimes this would involve the breaking of a light bulb or a drinking glass, the shards to be shared by the group as a means of sealing the pact—in blood.

Many of the girls told us that the consequences of not performing according to the expectations of the peer group in these events could be dire. The means of dealing with reluctant participants were varied and ingenious. They did not entail simple physical beatings, but rather took the form of some complex group-supported plot to place the girl in jeopardy. For example, they would plant some contraband in her room and then subtly arrange for a matron to find it. Such schemes were extremely difficult to detect. In many cases it would take months to unravel some bizarre plot apparently designed to portray the reluctant or unwilling participant as a serious institutional problem. In short: If you don't play, you pay.

Ritual and symbolism plays a part in many other self-mutilating behaviors. Many self-mutilating individuals explain their behavior in language laden with religious overtones and symbolism. These range from the facetious, "the devil made me do it," to the seriously disturbed, "God told me last night that I must be punished for my evil thoughts." Such reports have led some investigators to search for an understanding of the behavior by exploring the parallels in the sacred and secular traditions of ceremony and ritual. The literature on religious behavior describes numerous and severe acts of self-injury. For example, a recent case was reported of a young Brazilian man who walked on hot coals and ground glass, swallowed razors, screws, and light bulbs, and then inserted nails through his cheeks. He did so, presumably, as an act of faith in the powers of a long dead priest (*Newsweek*, February 27, 1978, p. 86).

Acts of cutting or flaying of the body for purification or atonement for sin or guilt are not just the subject matter of anthropologists studying the sub-incision rites of primitive tribes but are also found in reports of religious and cult ceremony in many developed countries.

There is often a quality of magical thinking in the cognitive processes of self-mutilators. Some not only attempt to atone for guilt through self-punishment but also actually ascribe supernatural or magical powers to their act. Clanon (1965), Asch (1971), and Crabtree (1967) have noted that their self-mutilating patients felt that their acts somehow purified their bodies, cleansed their blood, or eliminated poisons.

Christian theologians have addressed the issues of mutilation by adherence to the fundamental principle that man is custodian, not proprietor, of his physical being. Thus, disposal of bodily members, or other acts which serve to impair the body or its functions, must be guided by the principle of totality:

> By virtue of the principle of totality, by virtue of his right to use the services of his organism as a whole, the patient can allow individual

> parts to be destroyed or mutilated when and to the extent necessary for the good of his being as a whole. He may do so to ensure his being's existence and to avoid or . . . to repair serious and lasting damage which cannot otherwise be avoided or repaired. [Pius XII, cited in *New Catholic Encyclopedia*, 1967, p. 145]

Although this principle has provided useful guidelines for theologians in dealing with many contemporary medical issues ranging from castration to cosmetic surgery, its applicability to many of the practices of self-mutilators is problematic, controversial, and by no means clear.

The biblical exhortations ascribed to Jesus in the verses of Mark, chapter 9, outlines the principle of the sacrifice of the lesser good for the sake of the greater good:

> And if thy hand offend thee, cut it off: it is better for thee to enter into life maimed, than having two hands to go into hell, into the fire that shall never be quenched: . . .
>
> And if thy foot offend thee, cut it off: it is better for thee to enter halt into life, than having two feet to be cast into hell, into the fire that never shall be quenched: . . .
>
> And if thine eye offend thee, pluck it out: it is better for thee to enter into the kingdom of God with one eye, than having two eyes to be cast into the hell fire. [Mark, chapter 9: 43–48]

In brief, "whatever hinders entrance into the kingdom is a fatal liability" (*The Interpreter's Bible*, 1962, p. 792). The parts of the body, no matter how indispensable, are better sacrificed than left to become instruments of evil.

Biblical injuctions have been interpreted literally by self-mutilators. For example, Carson and Lewis (1971) describe a sixteen-year-old boy who, upon hearing a voice exhorting "if thy right eye offend thee, pluck it out," did precisely that. Investigators describing incidents of ocular self-enucleation performed while in a hallucinatory state report that the content of the hallucination is likely to have religious overtones and include instructions to remove the offending organ. (Goodhart and Savitsky, 1933; Hartman, 1925).

Other parts of the body have been severed or maimed where the act is endowed with religious significance or symbolism. Betts (1964) described a female patient who, identifying with Christ, drank her own blood and ate her own flesh as her personal communion.

Lubin (1961) has provided an extensive psychoanalytic interpretation of perhaps the most famous incident of self-mutilation, Vincent van Gogh's severing of his right ear. Lubin focuses on the religious symbolism of the act and the subsequent presentation of the mutilated organ to a prostitute (Rachel):

> In giving the mother surrogate, Rachel, a dead segment of his body, he symbolically repeats the scene on calvary after the crucifixion . . . When he presents it to Rachel, he in effect repeats the words of Jesus: "take, eat: this is my body." [P. 73]

It is even possible that his self-mutilation represented his attempt to model a ceremony that symbolizes the bravery and skill of a matador. Apparently van Gogh was intrigued by the ceremony in which the ear of the bull is excised and offered to a female spectator (Lubin, 1961).

Van Gogh's case is particularly noteworthy because it illustrates clearly the complexity of motivational forces which presumably are involved in an act of self-mutilation. Lubin's (1961) description of the psychoanalytic, postmortem explanations of van Gogh's behavior is in itself a classic example of the lack of reliability that characterizes post hoc historical reconstruction of the antecedents of self-mutilating acts. As Lubin has noted the ear cutting has been attributed to a myriad of motivational forces including castration fears, repressed homosexual impulses, and guilt. Van Gogh's psychological development has been described as masochistic. He apparently admired sick people, particularly those who had been maimed, and often used crippled individuals as models. His mutilatory behavior may have been related to auditory hallucinations which pained him, and he cut his ear off to remove the source of pain as he did his teeth when they bothered him. The ear, to some psychoanalytic theorists, symbolizes the penis (others claim it symbolizes the vagina, rectum, or mouth!). By cutting off the symbolic penis, van Gogh imagined that he might obtain the favor of his mother who wished him to be the opposite of a rough boy—helpless and vulnerable.

Some positors of plogglies have a proclivity for poetry

Psychobiological Determinants

It is tempting for the observer of the self-mutilating individual who is distressed by the apparent senselessness of such behavior to conclude, in an effort to provide himself with a feeling of reassurance, that the mutilator is "not one of us." We are somehow comforted by the fact that many mutilators are patients in psychiatric centers and thus different from the common folks, or are inmates in a correctional institution and, therefore, some sort of variant of human nature. "Nice folks don't carve" we say to ourselves as we attempt to separate ourselves from the self-mutilator. By assuming that there are plogglies which are responsible for self-mutilation, we are able to attribute blame to factors outside of our ordinary environment, and we can, thereby, distance ourselves from an offensive reality. An even more effective defense is to assume that there are plogglies which only affect particular types of people—people with specific vulnerabilities.

One way to do this is to attribute self-mutilation to some psychobiological factor. Unfortunately, no one has as yet discovered a gene for self-mutilation or presented convincing evidence of a hereditary factor in such behavior. However, the notion that a psychobiological determinant may be implicated in some forms of self-mutilation should not be lightly dismissed.

Self-mutilation may in some rather rare instances be a manifestation of the Cornelia de Lange syndrome (de Lange, 1933). This is clearly established clinical entity, a congenital disease characterized by retardation of physical and mental development, hirsutism and low birth weight, and distinguishing physical features such as excessively small face and head, long eyelashes, very thin and turned down lips, micromelia of the feet or hands, and, in many cases, deformities of the bones in the arms. Bryson, et al., (1971) and Shear et al., (1971) have reported a variety of self-mutilatory behaviors in Cornelia de Lange syndrome patients.

Self-mutilation seems to be characterisic of another organic disease: the Lesch-Nyhan syndrome (Lesch and Nyhan, 1964) in which a number of symptoms are found (mental retardation, choreoathetosis, hyperuricemia, gouty tophi of the fingers). As Bryson et al., (1971) have pointed out, the self-mutilating patient with Lesch-Nyhan syndrome engages in destructive and ferocious biting of the lips and fingers.

Reports are made in at least four articles of a metabolic defect which may be associated with self-mutilation (for example, Battle and Pollitt, 1964; Blacker and Wong, 1963; Hoefnagel et al., 1965; Segal et al., 1963). Korten et al., (1975) have recently described a case of self-mutilation in a patient with a chromosome aberration (49XXXXY). An earlier report of chromosonal abnormality was provided by Parker et al., (1970) in a case of 47XYY syndrome.

A high incidence of neurological impairment attributable to genetic or developmental defect has been reported by Bach-Y-Rita (1974) in his study of sixty-two habitually violent inmates in a California prison, 42 percent of whom had multiple scars on their body from self-inflicted wounds ("we frequently counted 75 to 100 scars on a particular patient"). Bach-Y-Rita noted that many of these men had a history of seizures, concussions, and loss of consciousness as children, and were "prone to perceptual disturbances." He concludes that there is a possibility of neurological impairment in such cases, but no further concrete evidence is provided.

Soeb (1948; reported in Davidson, 1962) has reported a case of self-enucleation in which an epileptic patient blinded himself with his fingernails in order to rid himself of his epilepsy. However, one cannot attribute the cause of this behavior directly to the epilepsy but only to the peculiar cognitive processes of this particular patient.

Finally, in discussing psychobiological determinants of self-mutilation, we should note the aberrant pain behavior of some schizophrenic children (for example, Goldfarb, 1958) and the apparent insensitivity of pain of many self-mutilating patients while they are injuring themselves. The possibility of a congenital agnosia (insensitivity) to pain (for example, Critchely, 1956) or a developed one (Money, Wolff, and Annecillo, 1972) may be associated with self-mutilating in some patients, but as in other psychobiological hypotheses, such conditions are unlikely to explain the mutilating behavior of very many mutilators.

Sex

We have not yet mentioned whether plogglies are male, female, or neuter. It is appropriate not to do so when discussing self-mutilating since many self-mutilators apparently are not quite sure whether they are male, female or neuter. According to some investigators, it is precisely this confusion of sexual identification which motivates them to injure themselves. For example, the genital self-mutilation of a thirty-nine-year-old housewife was attributed to the difficulties she had been having in accepting her role as a female. Her difficulties started at an early age when she began feeling that her mother had wanted to have a boy rather than a girl. They continued throughout her life and were reflected in her maintaining a male image in clothes and hairstyle, and in major difficulties she experienced in sexual adjustment. During five pregnancies, only two of which carried to term, she experienced what were described as bizarre symptoms, including inexplicable bleeding and alleged spontaneous abortions. It was suspected that many of her symptoms were the result of self-mutilation. The persistence of her gynecological problems led eventually to a hysterectomy; a conclusion whereby "she may have achieved her aims" (Goldney and Simpson, 1975). Two other cases of females whose behavior was viewed as symptomatic of active rejection of female identification are described by these investigators, who suggested the term *Caenis syndrome* to represent such cases. Caenis is a mythological female who, after being raped by Neptune, wished to cease being a female in order to avoid undergoing such an injury again.

Psychosexual confusion is seen as the motivational basis for the acts of many self-mutilating patients. Gardner and Gardner (1975), in a controlled study of the clinical features of twenty-two female patients who repeatedly cut themselves, noted a significantly higher incidence of psychosexual disorder among the cutting groups, who were more likely to be frigid or actively lesbian than their matched, noncutting controls. Blacker and Wong (1963) have indicated that sexual confusion of a long and intense type was a common element in their study of autocastration patients. Similar observations were made by Goldney and Simpson (1975) in cases of female genital self-mutilation, by Nelson and Grunebaum (1971) with wrist-slashers, and by Novotny (1972) and Siomopoulos (1974) with other types of repetitive self-cutting.

The sexual aspects involved in cases of genital self-mutilation probably appear reasonable to many of us. However, we may have difficulty with the analyses of other self-mutilations in sexual terms. According to Freudian psychoanalytic theorizing, excitation of the body of any kind, including that engendered by muscular stimuli and kinesthetic stimuli, is a potential source of sexual excitement. Pain itself can be highly sexual.

Slawson and Davidson (1964) reported the case of a female patient who bit off the tip of her tongue:

> She described her tongue as having an "urge to be bitten" . . . This urge was often more unpleasant than the excruciating pain experienced immediately after a bite. [P. 583]

Slawson and Davidson have interpreted this behavior as a "teeth-tongue" conflict where the teeth serve as the aggressive instrument of the mouth, the symbol of the vagina, carrying out the unconscious wish to destroy the threatening organ, the tongue, a symbolic penis. Thus, in the unconscious equation of tongue equals penis, and mouth equals vagina, "the biting of the tongue is at one time a sadistic attack on and an incorporation of an organ both feared and desired." [p. 587]

The equation suggested by Slawson and Davidson is derived from an argument for the psychical substitution of penis by the tongue and vagina by the mouth. They argue that the penis and the tongue are similar: "elongated organs usually flaccid . . . lengthened and stiffened on protrusion. [Both have] power of movement, moistness and slipperyness" [p. 586]. The mouth and the vagina are "cavities lined with soft, moist, sensitive mucosa surrounded by skeletal muscle under some degree of voluntary control" [p. 587].

The pain of the act is seen as a warning signal to avoid yielding to the pleasant sexual sensations which engender the ambivalence. Self-mutilation serves a defensive purpose.

Michael and Beck (1972) suggest that the tongue amputation of one of their patients could be understood, in part, as symbolic self-castration, by arguing that:

> The tongue is also used as a source of gratification by internal sucking, often unconsciously as a masturbatory equivalent. It is like having a built-in nipple, pacifier, or penis. [P.96]

Thus, by symbolic substitution, "our patient possibly saved his genitals by the amputation" (p. 98).

The interpretation of self-mutilation as symbolic substitution of parts of the body for sexual organs has received attention from numerous investigators. For example, Mintz (1964) describes a thirty-seven-year-old man who cooked and ate his fingers:

> He burned his index finger to a crisp and was able to withstand the pain. Then ate his distal and middle phalanx. He began to burn his wrist with the intention of eating his hand, but found that the wrist and the left axilla were much more difficult to burn and subsequently gave it all up. [P. 1017]

The eating of the finger (in this equation finger equals penis) reflected, according to Mintz, the gratification of forbidden homosexual impulses.

Self-cutting has been interpreted by many investigators as having a distinct sexual component such as symbolic self-castration (Brenman, 1952; Menninger, 1938; Michael and Beck, 1973; Novotny, 1972; Phillips and Alkan, 1961; Rado, 1933), a defense against sexual feelings (Nelson and Grunebaum, 1971), or a symbolic substitute for masturbation (Fenichel, 1945; Stekel, 1961; Siomopoulos, 1974).

Podvoll (1969) notes that high risk mutilation patients seem to suddenly cease these activities after revelations to a therapist of their masturbatory wishes, fellatio fantasies, or homoerotic thoughts. Burnham (1969) has noted that the climax of the cutting episode is analagous to masturbatory orgasm. Stekel (1961) noted that the cessation of masturbatory activities in certain patients coincided with an increase in suicidal gestures. Siomopoulos (1974) notes that:

> One may notice that both masturbation and self-cutting are forms of "self-abuse," being actions of the subject on his own body for purposes unacceptable or unjustified by common social standards. [P. 89]

Self-cutting, then, is interpreted as distorted autoerotic activity in which:

> The self-cutter opens up symbolically through her cutting multiple little female genitals on her skin, which becomes available for uninhibited touching, handling and all sorts of manipulations. [Siomopoulos, 1974, p. 90]

The etiology of self-cutting as an impulse neurosis is for Siomopoulos explained by the changing role of women in our culture. The dynamics of self-cutting reside in the mother's renunciation of maternal duties, producing excessive frustrations in the infant which must be compensated for by autoerotic fixation—"if she won't touch me-I'll have to do it myself."

Sexist plogglies are not uncommon.

Whereas many explanations cite sexual conflicts as motivational factors in self-mutilation, specific reference to oedipal conflict is surprisingly rare in the literature. However, Davidson (1962) does refer frequently to unresolved oedipal conflicts in his ocular self-enucleation subjects, some of whom, he suggests, removed their eyes in order to avoid incestuous or destructive urges toward their mother or father or to produce "mental immunity" from distressing sexual thoughts. Similarly, Stinnet and Hollender (1970) describe a compulsive eye banger who had suffered complete loss of vision in one eye and 60 percent loss in the other as a result of constantly battering the eyes. These incidents were said to have been precipitated by anxiety and guilt over erotic fantasies about his mother.

Archaic Biological Reflexes

The renowned psychoanalyst, Otto Fenichel, suggested that self-mutilatory behavior could be explained by an archaic biological reflex akin to that found in animals trying to escape from traps. Many animals who have had limbs ensnared have literally chewed off their limbs in order to escape. Similar acts of desperation, Fenichel reasons, are those in which humans sever or destroy parts of their body. By so doing they are sacrificing part of their body to preserve the remainder of their body. For example, it is by no means an uncommon practice for individuals infected with gangrene to self-amputate a limb in order to prevent the spread of gangrene throughout the body. It is not surprising that some investigators would see a parallel between such acts of survival and other self-mutilatory acts and to attempt to make sense out of such apparently bizarre behavior by assuming that the behavior has an adaptive or protective function for the mutilator.

There is an obvious parallel between Fenichel's psychoanalytic interpretation and a behavioristic account of masochism proposed by Skinner (1953) in which he suggested that organisms might deliberately "expose themselves to aversive stimulation if, by doing so, they avoid even more aversive consequences" (reported in Sandler, 1964, p. 201).

Death Wish

In view of the similarity of some forms of self-mutilation to suicidal behavior, and the fact that self-mutilation sometimes unintentionally leads to death, it is reasonable to expect that investigators would attempt to explain self-injury as a manifestation of a death wish (Ferenczi, 1956). A death wish is an aggressive instinct which, if expressed in direct unmodified form, would lead to the death of the person or of other people.

> It is well established that suicide is the result of murder wishes that have been directed from the objects of them in the other world and have been turned inward against the self. [Jones, 1938; cited in Hinsie, 1960, p. 176]

It is surprising that few investigators (for example, Ferenczi, 1956) have argued strongly for a death wish interpretation of self-mutilation. On the contrary, many investigators have concluded that the self-mutilator is not intent on dying and that his behavior actually is contraintentional to suicide. Of course, it is perfectly possible to interpret the absence of suicidal intent or the intention to avoid suicide as a symbolized death wish, a death wish in disguise, a reaction formation against a death wish.

Some plogglies have a mercurial quality.

Regression

Some self-mutilators appear to be preoccupied with their body. They view their skin as a primary, sometimes the only, source of satisfaction available to them. Some psychoanalytically oriented writers (Kafka, 1969; Pao, 1969; Podvoll, 1969) have suggested that the mutilator responds to his body as though it were a love object and have noted that the mutilator is like a child in this respect. They have reasoned that, faced with conflicts such as one encounters at puberty, the mutilator regresses to an earlier stage of development, to an earlier level of adaptation. In most instances, it is suggested, they regress to a preoedipal infantile stage during which satisfaction is obtained through tactile-kinesthetic stimulation. In a slight departure, Michael and Beck (1973) suggest that that the tongue-severing act of one of their patients could be seen as an attempt to regress to a preoedipal stage when he had a speech impediment which he blamed for separating him from his mother's affection.

Observations that we made of many of our Grandview mutilators would support the notion that there is a childlike quality in their behavior. Frequently these girls, like infants, appeared to be totally self-centered, unable to delay gratification of their needs, demanding of attention and preoccupied with their bodies and bodily processes. Whether they had regressed to this more primitive stage or had never advanced beyond it remained a moot point.

Existential Statement

Go ahead, slice yourself to ribbons; let's find out if you're alive or not.

–Kafka, 1969

Many of the mutilators at Grandview reported that before their self-injurious act they felt dead or empty. They seemed to be devoid of feeling, unreal, unable to distinguish themselves from other objects and unaware or unsure of the existence of their bodies.

Responding to similar comments by their patients, many investigators have concluded that self-mutilation is an existential statement, a means whereby the individual is able to confirm his existence. It has been described as an act which serves to reassure the individual that he is alive, that he has feelings, that he has an identity, and that he is indeed distinct from his surroundings. Collins (1965), for example, explains self-mutilation in a twenty-two-year-old head banger as an act designed to "maintain a self-identity through constant reinforcement of the perception of the extent of his body—a most primitive and basic level of existence" (p. 209).

In a symposium on self-mutilation, Gioviacchini (1956) talked about the adaptive function of pain which can help to develop "self-representation" or "facilitate individuation." He argues that patients who question whether they are alive or dead, asleep or awake, can reassure themselves by pain since "feeling is equated with life, non-feeling with non-existence. To feel reassuring that one is alive even if that feeling is pain" (p. 227). The obvious analogy is pinching ourselves to assure ourselves that we are awake. Self-mutilation can be viewed as confirmation of life. In a sense, life is imbued with meaning by confronting death. To bleed is to live.

Specific reference to a state of "depersonalization" is frequently made by psychodynamically oriented investigators. Depersonalization is the state or process of being dissolved, of losing one's identity. The depersonalized patient often has no sense of the reality of others or of his environment. The development of such an altered ego state as a precursor and presumed cause of self-mutilation is described in many reports (for example, Asch, 1971; Bach-Y-Rita, 1974; Bach-Y-Rita and Veno, 1974; Collins, 1965; Gardner and Gardner, 1975; Kafka, 1971; Miller and Bashkin, 1974; Pao, 1969; Podvoll, 1969; Roback et al., 1972; Rosenthal et al., 1972).

Kafka (1971) has described how the mutilator can treat his body as a transitional object which he can use as a means of differentiating external reality from internal reality. Cutting the body, he reasons, can allow the patient to clear up the ambiguity between what is self and what is not-self. The body serves as a point of reference.

Miller and Bashkin (1974) have suggested that the self-mutilatory act is the culmination of a sequence of specific events which start with some frustrating experience which leads the patient to feel totally rejected or abandoned as well as overwhelmingly angry. The rage, it is suggested, leads to depersonalization. Self-mutilation enables the patient to escape depersonalization and to discharge rage and fear (Asch, 1971).

Rosenthal et al. (1972) have argued that the self-cutting in their patients represented attempts at reintegration when they have depersonalized in reaction to being unable to cope with specific feelings. They describe the cutting as a "primitive way of combatting the feeling of unreality and emptiness." "Look, self, I can feel pain," or "I bleed; therefore, I am alive," or "I do have insides; I can see them" (p. 51). They report that twenty-three of twenty-five incidents of self-cutting occurred while the patients were depersonalized.

In a similar vein Asch (1971) has called a group of promiscuous adolescent female patients who frequently have scratched their wrists "as-if girls." He suggests that their behavior is symptomatic of a state of anhedonia, which is a primitive state of depression characterized by passivity and submissiveness (with sporadic destructive rage outbursts), poor object relations, and anxiety about possible separation from others. Such patients have little valid affect and do not know what they feel. They also are highly labile emotionally, given to rapid mood swings, and feel hopeless, empty, dead, or bored.

Asch notes that they are narcissistic but have only a vague perception of themselves. When they feel they are being rejected, they become overwhelmed by rage and then depersonalize. The sight of their blood relieves the terrifying fear of the depersonalization in which they are unable to differentiate themselves from their environment.

> There was too much white, white nurses, white doctors, white sheets, white walls. It was such a relief to cut and see the red blood appear. [P. 612]

As Bach-Y-Rita (1974) and Bach-Y-Rita and Veno (1974) have noted, the assumption that depersonalization is a factor in the causation of self-mutilation is consistent with the generally accepted conclusion that self-mutilation often occurs without pain. The depersonalization reaction may, in fact, represent an altered state of consciousness in which the perception of pain is considerably reduced. Interestingly, most patients report the absence of pain during the act, but many do experience pain immediately following. This is consistent with the notion of an altered state. When reintegration occurs the patient is no longer in the altered state of depersonalization and, therefore, is again able to experience pain.

Based on the assumption that self-mutilation represents the patient's attempt to feel something, at least one psychiatric hospital has considered the use of medication as a means of helping patients to experience feelings without having to resort to self-mutilation (Roback et al., 1972). The effectiveness of the medication as a means of eliminating depersonalization and, thereby, warding off further self-injurious behavior has not yet been adequately demonstrated. On the other hand, the effectiveness of self-mutilation as a means of eliminating depersonalization has been clearly demonstrated. It is a highly effective form of adaptation which brings immediate beneficial results to a terrifying state.

Plea for Help

Suicide has often been described as a *cry for help*, a means of forcing people to recognize the suffering that the individual is experiencing, an indirect but dramatic way of communicating that the individual needs aid. The act is a graphic portrayal of the pain that he is suffering. Self-mutilation may be similarly motivated as a means of stimulating others to come to the rescue (Bostic, 1973; Offer and Barlow, 1960; Alderson, 1974).

Manipulation

Some acts of self-mutilation are rather perverse strategies by which the individual manipulates people into satisfying his wishes. Such manipulations have a high probability of success. They often can be much more effective than direct requests or demands. The consequences of not listening to a mutilator can be dramatic, dire, and highly visible. Because it has been culturally ingrained in most of us to be responsive, kind, and considerate to people who are in pain, the patient readily has us over a moral barrel by making it clear that if we don't do what he wants he will mutilate himself. Implicit in his threat is the fact that he can make us responsible for his actions. The manipulative mutilator can dangle his attendants on strings through his "emotional blackmail" (Brenman, 1952). He can obtain tremendous power by his threats. To call his bluff is to invite the mutilator not only to carry out his threat but also to increase the severity of his destructive behavior. To give into his demands is likely to encourage greater and more frequent demands. There is no apparent solution to this form of blackmail, which can become the bane of the institutional administrator. It is perhaps a greater threat in an institutional setting, because it is in such places almost by definition that we adopt the view that we, not the patient, are responsible for the patient's behavior—a view that makes us easy targets for manipulation.

Manipulators have used many self-injurious acts quite deliberately and intentionally to their advantage in many ways: to obtain attention, to get access to therapy, to win transfer to a more preferred location (Johnson, 1975), to influence social agencies to cater to their needs (Morgan, Barton, and Pottle, 1976), even to wile their way out of institutions and back again. The well-known hospital hobo (also referred to as malingering or having the Munchausen syndrome) moves around the country living at the expense of the hospitals which admit him and is often treated for injuries and illnesses which he has self-induced as a rather unorthdox way of earning his keep.

Often the mutilator's physical behavior is at variance with his verbal behavior. Many carvers at Grandview spent a large part of their waking hours lamenting their plight at being confined in a training school which they condemned in startlingly blasphemous language. But they continued to carve themselves in order that the administrators would refuse to allow them to leave. The adept mutilator, through behavior or threats, can literally control the resources of institutions or social agencies or families or any individual with a modicum of humanity (Ferster, 1968; Smolev, 1971). It is, in an important way, a highly adaptive behavior.

The literature is replete with examples of self-mutilations which have been explained as manipulations employed by individuals lacking a repertoire of alternative behaviors which can gain them the ends they seek, or by individuals faced with environmental conditions which prevent them from exercising coping behaviors (Bach-Y-Rita, 1974; Bach-Y-Rita and Veno, 1974; Claghorn and Beto, 1967; Cookson, 1977; Cox and Klinge, 1976; Crabtree, 1967; Ferster, 1968; Jacobson and Tribe, 1972; Nelson and Grunebaum, 1971; Smolev, 1971).

Podvoll (1969) provides a description of the attendant environment of the self-mutilating patient with an administrator threatening resignation, previously collegial social workers and other staff engaged in bitter squabbles as a result of the stress, and exhaustion engendered by continuous patient-precipitated crises, and, simultaneously, a serious custody confrontation between the patient's parents before a divorce court.

Risk Taking

When they deliberately cut veins, sever arteries, swallow glass, or otherwise engage in self-mutilatory behavior, individuals may not intend to kill themselves or even incapacitate themselves, but they often, wittingly or not, are incurring a considerable risk of death. Some mutilators may actually injure themselves for just that reason—to take a risk. Such acts may reflect simple poor judgment or judgment impaired by overingestion of alcohol (Frankel et al., 1976), or an alcohol or drug-induced increased willingness to engage in risk behavior (Sjoberg, 1969). Risk taking may also be a "macho" response designed to provide temporary nourishment to self-esteem. It may be a way of enlivening an otherwise lackluster existence, an act designed for excitement. It may also be a way of engendering a response in other people by frightening them by the very daring of the risk. People who take risks often attract a considerable audience. An audience, real or imaginary, can create the necessary stimulus for the self-mutilator to indulge in grandstanding. Risk taking is, in effect, gambling. Often the mutilator gambles that his act will not have serious consequences, that some providential agent will intervene to rescue him. He will even gamble that the pleasure derived from the actual act of mutilating or from its consequence will be worth whatever discomfort it will cause him. Self-mutilators may be tempting fate, testing the kindness of God or luck to see whether they are to be approved or rejected. They may be gamblers, just as Lester and Lester (1971) have suggested is the case in suicide, where every act is a "gamble with death."

Attention Seeking

The most prevalent explanation of self-mutilation in the literature we reviewed was that it is an act conceived and perpetrated with a view to obtaining attention (for example, Bachman, 1972; Claghorn and Beto, 1967; Cookson, 1977; Crabtree, 1967; Cox and Klinge, 1976; Nelson and Grunebaum, 1971; Romanczyk and Goren, 1975; Offer and Barlow, 1960; Rosenthal et al., 1972).

McNeil and Vance (1978) describe the acts of prisoners in solitary confinement units—the "holes"—of several Canadian penitentiaries (including the infamous forty-four cell "penthouse" of the British Columbia Penitentiary):

> To get attention, they occasionally set themselves afire, or slash themselves with razor blades. Arms and torsos are covered with the scars of the blades. [P. 18]

Attention is often in short supply in institutions, but it is remarkable how plentiful it becomes when someone mutilates himself. Sometimes the attention seeking of the mutilator is so blatant that one might wonder whether the additional staff that institutional managers often introduce in response to an incident of self-mutilation might be more effectively assigned to provide attention to the potential mutilator before he resorts to mutilation. On many occasions at Grandview additional staff were introduced to provide round-the-clock supervision of a girl for several days after she had carved. Why not use this help proactively rather than reactively? At Grandview there were at least three reasons: (1) it was easier to justify additional expenditure when a crisis was involved; (2) since so many girls were potential carvers, providing personal supervision to the degree that would have been required would involve a monumental increase in the budget (the staff:girl ratio was already better than 1:1), and (3) the attention needs of many mutilators appeared to be insatiable. We came to believe that the more staff that were available to the girls, the more self-mutilation would occur. The maxim for some of the girls seemed to be, the larger the audience, the deeper the cut.

Self-mutilation is a singularly effective way of gaining attention. In most instances it is 100 percent successful. Even the best trained staff are usually unable to avoid responding to the mutilator in a well-intentioned effort to comfort them or reprimand them. If they are able to withold such responses, there are few individuals who can fail to portray their distress, revulsion, or horror when they see the damage the mutilator has done to his body. Recognizing that mutilating is designed to yield attention, many people have attempted to withhold their attention when the mutilator injures himself; in response the patient merely increases the frequency or severity of his act to the point where even the most stoic observer yields.

One of the major difficulties with the attention seeking of self-mutilation in institutional settings is that it works; it yields results. Anything that yields results in institutions takes on an aura of importance and inevitably will lead to others becoming interested; it will be imitated. At Grandview we had many imitators, girls who were not serious about engaging in self-mutilating behavior, at least not at first. However, after a time, they would see the results of the other girls' carving. Their repugnance for the behavior would begin to vie with their need for attention, especially when they saw the attention that their models' behavior elicited.

Iatrogenic

The role of the therapist or staff in the unintentional triggering of a self-mutilatory act in their patients must not be overlooked. Most reports on self-mutilation stress the importance of rejection or the separation of parents or loved ones as immediate precursors of self-mutilation. However, few make any mention that rejection of the mutilator by the institutional staff may be just as likely to engender a self-mutilating incident. As we learned only too well with the adolescents at Grandview, the relationship between the mutilator and his therapist is often highly tenuous at the best of times and can often explode as a result of some innocuous event which the mutilator perceives or misconstrues as rejection or condemnation. Many self-mutilating acts have been a reaction to a distressing encounter in therapy or on the ward when an unsuspecting staff member has unintentionally frustrated a mutilating patient. Frequently self-mutilation occurs immediately following a therapy session, perhaps as a result of a stressful discussion or of feelings of loneliness that some patients feel when they contrast their social involvement on the ward with the intensity of their involvement in therapy. Therapy per se may be iatrogenic as, for instance, when patients mutilate themselves in order to obtain their therapist's attention or in order to somehow justify or make sense out of their involvement in therapy—"I'm in therapy, therefore I must act as a patient." Some patients may mutilate themselves because nothing else they do gets them so much attention from their therapists.

> If I came through your office door covered with blood and still bleeding, you'd probably just sit there and ask me what I was thinking about before I cut. [Podvoll, 1969, p. 215]

At Grandview, the girls often tested the limits with their therapists. They frequently teased therapists with statements like: "What would you do if I carved?" "I think I'm going to cut myself tonight," or, "Don't be surprised if you see me differently tomorrow," and so on. Often these were worded in a way that they ensured that the therapist would join in the game and persuade the girl not to carve.

Sometimes a therapist would defuse a girl with humorous banter:

Patient: It's getting to be too much—I've decided—tonight's the night—I'll cut myself tonight.

Therapist (looking at his watch): I'm afraid you can't, not tonight—it's Tuesday —there's no nurse on duty tonight.

Patient (thoughtfully): You're right—OK, but wait until next time.

It requires outstanding clinical acumen to recognize when it is appropriate and safe for the therapist to respond in such a way. Many professionals who have worked with mutilators can recall incidents in which a patient who had been engaged in a light-hearted exchange in an afternoon session was found bathed in blood several hours later.

Podvoll (1969) has clearly articulated the role that staff and therapists can play in maintaining self-mutilation in their patients. For example, by identifying the patient in terms of his symptoms, they may establish expectancies which become self-fulfilling prophecies that the symptoms will be displayed. The patient can come to feel that his symptoms are all he possesses, and he clings obstinately to them as his only source of identity. The folly of labeling was clearly demonstrated to us at Grandview when the staff, in an honest effort to give the girls improved protection, developed a carvers list so that all the staff would know to be vigilant in supervising these girls. The girls lived up to their reputation. The list significantly augmented the problem to the point where it was really unnecessary to have a list: the carvers were readily identified by everyone by their scars.

Retaliation

Many of the explanations of self-mutilation are derived from statements made by self-mutilators who after their act have been asked why they injured themselves. Far more illuminating would be knowledge of what the mutilator says to himself just before he mutilates or while he is in the act of mutilating—data about his internal dialogue before it is distorted by time or the demands of an interview which requires him to explain his behavior. Fortunately (or perhaps unfortunately), we were, because of our crisis-intervention role, often able to talk to the girls immediately after they had carved themselves and, embarassingly, immediately before they carved themselves, at which time we would try to talk the girl out of carving (usually unsuccessfully). Our experience led us to agree with other investigators (Johnson, 1973; Nelson and Grunebaum, 1971) who have suggested that some self-mutilation represents retaliatory behavior. The individual, either because he lacks the skills to retaliate in a direct manner or because his environment prevents it, may use self-mutilation as an indirect means of getting back at someone. For example, by mutilating he may create difficulty for a prison official who will be taken to task for failing to adequately discharge his responsibility to control his inmates. "Now look what you've made me do," "I'll show you," I told you I'd do it if you . . ." "You'll be sorry now," and many other similar statements were frequently expressed by the Grandview mutilators.

Self-mutilation in the hands of a vindictive person can represent, literally, raw power. By hurting himself, he can have a very effective means of hurting others. As a response to perceived ill-treatment or injustice the act has symbolic significance. The harm that is done to the mutilator's body mirrors the harm that has been done to him: "See how badly you've treated me?" It places the burden for the act on the person they see as the provocateur. It is a highly efficacious means of playing on the guilt feelings of the person whom the mutilator views as the perpetrator. Apart from the blood and scars, it is often difficult to determine who is the victim. The retaliative self-mutilator assumes that some people care enough to be affected.

Frustration

Institutions generally provide both explicit and implicit sanctions against aggressive outbursts of temper or explosive rage. Physical or even verbal expressions of frustration are likely to be prohibited for the good order of the institution. Ironically, the environment which prevents the expression of emotional responses to frustration also foster the frustration by virtue of the restrictions and controls it establishes.

The frustrated resident of an institution often has very little opportunity to respond vigorously to frustration and may have to suppress the aggressive impulses that his frustration engenders. In some instances he may vent his frustration by self-mutilation.

Many acts of self-mutilation may be responsive to environmental restrictions and frustration (e.g., Bach-Y-Rita, 1974; Bach-Y-Rita and Veno, 1974; Ballinger, 1971; McKerracher, Loughane, and Watson, 1968; Panton, 1962). The restrictions of the institutional milieu may be particularly problematic for the self-mutilator who may have low frustration tolerance and inadequate impulse control (Novotny, 1972).

In a way, self-mutilation may be a more effective means of venting frustration in an institution than is an outward explosive reaction, a direct confrontation with a frustrating staff member, or an attempt to eliminate or alter the environmental source of the frustration. Whereas the direct expression of frustration may have such aversive consequences as isolation, verbal rebuke, restrictions of privilege, and the like, reacting to frustration by self-mutilation is more likely to engender humane treatment, sympathy, succorance, extra attention, and special consideration by the staff, who may react supportively out of genuine concern, guilt, or a realistic fear that they will be further embarassed by their apparent inability to manage the institution. Ironically, self-mutilation may be far more disruptive to institutional decorum than is an outward display of frustration.

The frustration of living in the institution may be matched by the frustration of having to leave the institution. Anticipating departure from an institution as one's incarceration draws to an end may be a highly stressful experience for many residents. They often view with some fear the prospects of leaving a state of dependency in which many of their needs are met and having to adapt to a new environment and terminate relationships which have provided security for months or years. Many clinicians working in institutional settings learn that the few weeks before departure are very troubling times for many patients and have witnessed the apparent deterioration in the behavior of patients who had been making satisfactory progress.

This prerelease phenomenon was clearly demonstrated by some of the girls at Grandview who, after months of exemplary behavior, indulged in apparently senseless acts of vandalism and self-mutilation soon after learning they had earned their graduation from the institution. In noninstitutional settings similar incidents have been reported in patients frustrated by therapists who have decided to terminate treatment after concluding that the client's problems were resolved (Miller and Bashkin, 1974).

Frustration has also been suggested as one of the factors involved in the wrist slashers described by Nelson and Grunebaum (1971). These patients apparently had never learned how to express their feelings verbally and used self-mutilation as a means of discharging their feelings of constriction.

Contagion/Coercion/Conformity

The epidemic quality of self-mutilation, particularly within institutionalized female populations, has been noted by several investigators (for example, Cookson, 1977; Johnson, 1973; Matthews, 1968; McKerracher, Loughane, and Watson, 1968).

It may be that the epidemic is more metaphorical than actual. Although there may be psychobiological determinants of some instances of self-mutilation, it is unlikely that they can account for the fact that rashes of self-mutilating behavior are often apparently triggered by a single incident. A social contagion factor (Offer and Barlow, 1960) could account for outbreaks of self-mutilating incidents. Many mutilators may simply be imitating models who are seen to be obtaining rewards such as attention or status from their acts (Crabtree and Grossman, 1974),

Particularly in correctional settings, self-mutilation may be a clearly communicated way for an inmate to obtain status in an antiestablishment culture; a socially approved way of opposing administration-proscribed normative behaviors. More broadly, self-mutilation may be part of an initiation rite analogous to the initiatory self-mutilations in primitive cultural groups. Scars from self-mutilatory behavior may, of course, signify group membership and serve as identity badges similar to tatoos. In many instances at Grandview, girls were specifically coerced into carving themselves in order to avoid ostracism or in order to prove their allegiance to the group, or to demonstrate the depth of their affection for a girl friend who was threatening to reject her. In many cases the girls carved as part of a group agreement, party, or contract. Carving parties were not rare, and those who refused to participate did so at risk. At times it appeared that girls carved simply because it was fashionable to do so.

Matthews (1968) has reminded us of group-endorsed practices of self-injurious behavior among monks in the Middle Ages involving flagellation, prostration, and starvation. Group-supported outbreaks of self-mutilation have also been stimulated as a means of political protest. A recent example of this phenomenon is the incident at a Kansas State Penitentiary in which several inmates severed their Achilles tendons. In Canada, an investigation of the Canadian penitentiary system heard evidence:

> concerning guards who have given known slashers razor blades and taunted them to slash themselves. On occasion the inmates have done as they were told. At B.C. Penitentiary at least nine inmates in one range slashed themselves on Christmas Eve 1976 after a guard left two razor blades in a cell and told them to "have a Merry Christmas and a slashing New Year" [MacGuigan, 1977, p. 44]

During the preparation of this work we received a number of anecdotal personal communications citing examples of self-mutilation epidemics by prisoners in, for example, an Israeli prison and a Canadian jail.

In spite of the frequency of references in the literature to epidemics of self-mutilation there is really very little concrete evidence of such phenomena. Matthews' (1968) systematic analysis traced the communication process presumed to underly the spread of self-injury in an adolescent unit. He was able to employ sociometric analysis to reconstruct the path of what he described as an epidemic of self-injury in a unit of twenty-five emotionally disturbed adolescents. One might question the appropriateness of the term *epidemic* in this instance since less than half the group, eleven cases, mutilated. Moreover, the incidents were spread over an eleven-month period. However, Matthews has shown clearly how social factors (contagion, conformity) can function in the spread of this behavior. Interestingly, one of his staff members "felt much attracted to the behavior and wanted to try it"!

We should note that the fact that there is little evidence to support the claims of epidemics may reflect, not the lack of validity of these claims, but the tendency of observers of such phenomena to refrain from reporting their observations. Self-mutilation is a taboo topic for many administrators. Reports may be actively suppressed or censored by those who do not wish to publicize the fact that such behaviors occur in their setting. To acknowledge that an institution is experiencing an epidemic of self-mutilation may be perceived by some as equivalent to admitting that the staff have lost control.

Our experience at Grandview convinced us that whereas self-mutilation may or may not have epidemic qualities it certainly has a cyclical quality. By carefully recording the occurrence of incidents of a variety of institutional offenses (for example, assault, AWOL, vandalism) including self-mutilation, we were able to determine that there was a pattern to the self-mutilating behavior in that institution. Specifically, the incidence of self-mutilation ("acting-in" behavior) increased when the frequency of the other misbehaviors ("acting-out" behaviors) decreased. However, rather than viewing the increase in self-mutilation in epidemic terms or in terms of specifically communicated in-group sanctions we viewed the outbreaks as a reflection of opportunity. When, for example, institutional security measures were tightened following a high incidence of abscondance (as happened very frequently) the girls, having less of an opportunity to escape, would carve instead.

Depression

Lubin (1961), in his extensive analysis of the ear-severing act of the artist Vincent van Gogh, has suggested that he was apparently severely depressed at the time. He was depressed by many things but particularly by the prospective marriage of his brother who would thereby be lost to him. Lubin has noted that the act occurred at Christmas—a time when depression is frequently experienced. McNeil and Vance (1978) describe a group of inmates whose "despair was made manifest over the Christmas holidays when a number . . . . slashed their arms" (p. 54).

As Cookson (1977) has mentioned, it is difficult to understand "why depression should be relieved by further pain" (p. 333), but depression is among the most common of the motives listed by patients to explain their acts, and most investigators have consistently reported that in a large proportion of cases mutilators are depressed just before they mutilate (Battle and Marshall, 1952; Blacker and Wong, 1963; Claghorn and Beto, 1967; Davidson, 1962; Jarvis et al., 1976; Offer and Barlow, 1960; Ryback, 1971; Siomopoulos, 1974). Such acts seem, at least on the surface, to have little instrumental value for the depressed person. Their depression is often reinstated when they later view the damage they have done to their body. We might speculate that cutting has some value akin to electroconvulsive (shock) therapy, but as in shock therapy we cannot clearly identify the process. If the depression is a consequence of guilt or anger, it may be that the self-mutilatory act appeases guilt or enables ventilation of anger through a punishing attack on the self.

An unusual rationale for the depression-mutilation link has been proposed by Rosenthal et al., (1972). They suggest that by mutilating, the patient counteracts the feeling of being overwhelmed. He takes action against himself which enables him to feel that he is in control.

Tension Relief

It is difficult for people to comprehend how anyone can deliberately set about to mutilate their body. It is more difficult for most of us to comprehend how they can do so without feeling any pain. Totally incomprehensible to most of us is the fact that many mutilators actually enjoy their experience. The act of cutting the skin has been described by self-cutters as an exquisitely pleasurable sensation (Evans, 1967; Kessel, 1966; Rosenthal et al., 1972; Stengel and Cook, 1958). Asch (1971) described a patient who, after cutting her wrists: "lay back on the bathroom floor, sensuously enjoying the experience. She felt progressively euphoric and comfortable as the 'black blood' oozed out" (p. 615). Similarly the rhythmical repetitive act of banging is frequently described by children as calming or soothing, "a relaxational expedient before falling asleep" (Gesell and Ilg, 1943).

Many Grandview carvers told us that preceding their mutilation they experienced a building up of tension often unrelated to any identifiable distressing thoughts or stressful events. Carving brought about an immediate diminution of tension and a warm pleasant feeling of relaxation. Many equated the experience to orgasm. Experiences like those described by the Grandview girls are experienced by many self-mutilators (Collins, 1965; Cookson, 1977; Claghorn and Beto, 1967; Crabtree and Grossman, 1974; Gardner and Gardner, 1975; Miller and Bashkin, 1974; Nelson and Grunebaum, 1971; Novotny, 1972; Offer and Barlow, 1960; Podvoll, 1969; Siomopoulos, 1974). Self-mutilation may be a rather unorthodox means of discharging tension or lowering anxiety. It may even be a means of achieving some sort of homeostatic resolution. It may very well be a means of discharging tension, particularly for those who lack more adaptive means either because of situational restrictions or because they have a limited behavioral repertoire.

Escape

We have already noted those behavioral explanations which view self-mutilation as an instrumental act which is acquired as a means of obtaining rewards or as a means of avoiding greater discomfort than is likely to ensue from the self-mutilation itself. Many investigators, without suggesting a conditioning perspective, simply view self-mutilation as a reaction to stress, conflict, fear, or guilt which may be temporary, situational, or characteristic of the person's environment for a long time.

Ballinger (1970), Jarvis et al. (1976), and Ferrence and Johnson (1974) have discussed self-mutilation in terms of a reaction to specific stressful events or more general or pervasive stressful conditions such as unemployment, illness, bereavement, marital problems, or change of domicile. It may be a reaction to the stresses of institutional life (Jarvis et al., 1976; Johnson, 1973). In prison settings it may be a response to fear; a means of avoiding attack from other inmates (Johnson, 1973; Clanon, 1965) or guards (McNeil and Vance, 1978). Self-mutilation often leads to an inmate being placed in protective custody to decrease the risk of further mutilation. By mutilating himself the prisoner can escape from the other inmates in such a way as not to appear to be "copping out" by asking for official help—an action which would lead to even greater hostility from his fellow inmates (Clanon, 1965).

The self-mutilation of some psychiatric patients has been explained as their way of avoiding loss of control of their fantasy life; a way of maintaining contact with reality (Offer and Barlow, 1960). One report describes a patient who blinded herself to escape a troubling hallucination (Davidson, 1962). It has also been seen as a means of avoiding overwhelming dependency on a therapist. Interestingly, some patients develop extreme possessiveness with respect to the objects they use to mutilate themselves and treat them like security blankets (Podvoll, 1969). One dependency is substituted for another.

Prisoners and soldiers have mutilated themselves as a means of avoiding distasteful work or unpleasant assignments or fear-provoking situations (e.g., Claghorn and Beto, 1967; Johnson, 1973). McNeil and Vance (1978) describe an inmate who had been a witness to a prior prison death. Confined in solitary and fearing some of the guards would kill him, he "slashed himself . . . . requiring 180 stitches" in order to escape from the direct access and control of these guards.

Dramatic examples of an individual mutilating herself in order to avoid activities or situations which are distressful are those cases in which females have mutilated their genitalia apparently in order to avoid sexual activity (for example, Goldfield and Glick, 1970; Simpson, 1973). Self-mutilation has also been explained in some cases as an attempt to avoid pregnancy or to terminate pregnancy (Simpson, 1973).

Finally, self-injurious acts may be perpetrated in order to bring about simple change. The patient may seek only an interruption in his life or a change in his environment (Cookson, 1977). Feeling trapped by monotony or various stresses, he may act in what appears to be an irrational manner simply to "get out of it" (Kessel, 1966). The withdrawal need not be as complete as it is in suicide. The change in the person's environment which follows a self-mutilation act is often abrupt, dramatic, and extreme. Self-mutilation is a powerful way to motivate other people to take action.

Drug-Related

Attempted and completed suicide involving the use of drugs has been well documented. Drugs may be involved in self-destructive behavior in at least two ways: (1) suicide may be attempted by the use of drugs, or (2) a drug-induced state may engender a suicide attempt. It is common for epidemiologists to include in their data on suicidal behavior or on self-injurious behaviors those behaviors which are not necessarily intended as suicide. Accordingly, it is not possible to determine the prevalence of drug-induced self-mutilatory behavior. Clearly there are many cases in which individuals have ingested drugs in an act of self-mutilation, and there are many instances where self-mutilatory behavior is triggered by a drug-induced state in which, for example, judgment is impaired, pain perception reduced, or fantasies stimulated. The dramatic case of self-enucleation reported by Carson and Lewis (1971) and noted in chapter 3, involved a young male who had been using drugs for two years (LSD, marijuana, methadrine) and enucleated during a high induced by a number of nasal inhalers.

Alcohol can also be involved in self-mutilating behavior. For example, Ryback (1971) has described the case of a thirty-two-year-old man who lacerated both wrists with a razor blade during a prolonged period of alcohol consumption. Interestingly, in this case, the subject was amnesic of the event and appears to have cut himself in an alcohol-produced dissociated state.

Johnson et al. (1975), in their epidemiological study in the city of London, Ontario, found that 50 percent of male self-injury cases and approximately 25 percent of the female cases were heavy drinkers. Drugs were implicated in 85 percent of all of the self-injuries. Because self-injury was broadly defined, it is not possible to extricate from their data the number of self-mutilating incidents in which drug use was involved.

Obviously, there are unresolved questions as to whether the alcohol or drugs directly engender self-mutilating behavior or merely decrease the potential self-mutilator's inhibition against self-mutilation.

Socioeconomic

Epidemiological investigations (for example, Bancroft et al., 1975) have found that reported self-injurious behavior is related to socioeconomic conditions. For example, rates are exceptionally high in teenage wives and single, divorced, or widowed women age twenty-four to thirty-five years; whereas the highest rate for men is in the thirty-five to forty-five-year age group. Rates are much higher in urban than in rural areas. Type of occupation is also a factor. In males, personal service workers, and semi-skilled or unskilled manual workers have the highest rates. Among females the highest rates are among nonmanual, or semi-skilled manual workers "ancillary to professional workers" (especially nurses). The incidence is highest in the lower social classes and in those who have a low degree of job involvement and satisfaction.

These relationships not only may be correlative but also may actually point to a causal link between socioeconomic factors and self-injury. However, because self-injury is so broadly defined in most epidemiological studies (most include incidents of self-poisoning or attempted suicide), it is not possible to determine their significance in self-mutilation.

Deprivation

A significant proportion of the Grandview carvers attributed their destructive acts to a feeling of boredom. These girls were able to feel bored even when surrounded by activities in which they would be welcome participants. Our staff spent many frustrating hours trying to encourage the girls to take part in recreational activities such as sports, hobbies, drama—anything! But most of the time the girls were content to do nothing. They seemed quite happy to be bored and much preferred to complain about a lack of activities than to participate in them. They seemed to have an insatiable appetite for demanding more activities and a remarkable proclivity for refusing to participate when their demands were met. "Nothing to do" was the continual lament, "boring" the chorus. Carving became a preferred way of relieving their self-imposed boredom.

Other investigators (Asch, 1971; Ballinger, 1971; McKerracher, Loughane, and Watson, 1968) have reported that boredom was a factor in their self-mutilating patients. Ballinger seems to relate boredom to environmental restrictions of institutional life, but in Grandview the number of activities which were made available during some phases of our intervention program provided these girls with far more recreational possibilities than are usually available to adolescents. Still they were bored; still they carved.

McKerracher, Loughane, and Watson (1968) reported that self-injury in their institution tended to occur on weekends when the patients had less to do. However, we found no evidence to support such a result among the Grandview mutilators, nor did Cookson (1977) in his study of self-injury among women at the Holloway Prison. Cookson reports that boredom contributed very little to self-mutilation with his subjects. However, examination of his data reveals that close to 70 percent of the self-injuries occurred in cells. Cells can be rather boring places in which to spend one's leisure time. So can institutions—even institutions like Grandview with bountiful opportunities for recreation. One has to keep in mind that many of our girls had been raised during their early adolescent years on a diet of unrestricted sex, alcohol, and drugs. Crochetting and baseball were rather pale substitutes.

Mutilators have been referred to as "stimulation seekers," and their self-injurious behavior has been attributed to conditions of stimulous deprivation (Asch, 1971; Bach-Y-Rita, 1974; Bach-Y-Rita and Veno, 1974; Money, Wolff, and Annecillo, 1972). Green (1968) has reported finding in the histories of schizophrenic self-mutilating children evidence of parental withdrawal and understimulation. He has conjectured that the child may mutilate himself in order to obtain parental contact even in the form of the kinesthetic stimulation which comes from physical punishment.

One particularly intriguing possibility in explaining self-mutilation is the hypothesis that attributes such behavior to sensorimotor or social deprivation in early life. There is some evidence to support the view that early childhood perceptual or social deprivation may be a precursor of maladaptive behavior in later life (Bowlby, 1952; Spitz, 1945; Spitz and Wolf, 1946). Support for this view is provided by studies of nonhuman primates which have been experimentally reared under conditions depriving them of contact with their mothers or other members of their species. Typically, these social isolates are raised in bare wire cages which allow them to see other animals and to smell and hear them, but prevent any physical contact between them—no touching, sucking, or somatosensory stimulation of any kind. A high frequency of self-mutilatory behavior in later life, particularly self-biting, has been observed in such socially deprived animals (Harlow, 1964; Harlow and Suomi, 1970; Mitchel, 1975).

Although they present no evidence that sensory deprivation actually occurred in the history of their patients, Money, Wolff, and Annecillo (1972), Bach-Y-Rita (1974) and Bach-Y-Rita and Veno (1974), do draw our attention to evidence which might support the notion of a specific link between early childhood stimulus deprivation and later self-injurious behavior. They point out that conditions which have been noted in the early life of self-mutilating patients or experimentally induced in primates are very similar to those which are reported in the early life of individuals with indifference or insensitivity to pain—specifically sensorimotor and social deprivation.

Their review of the evidence from the literature in this area is persuasive if not entirely conclusive. It is an intriguing possibility which requires further investigation, particularly in the form of longitudinal studies. In fact, we might be well advised to examine the possibility that any condition of intense or prolonged sensorimotor or social deprivation may put the individual at risk for self-mutilation. As we have noted, a significant proportion of the self-mutilating incidents in our cases occurred while the girls were in solitary confinement or restricted to their rooms. Although self-mutilation is not just an institutional syndrome, the unusually high frequency of self-mutilation in socially isolating and restricting environments such as institutions is not likely to be mere happenstance.

Response to the Body

When one runs out of plogglies by which to explain self-mutilation, it is always possible to blame the body for actions which are taken against it or at least to locate the causality in the body itself. In the literature there are many explanations which are offered by investigators or patients in which blame is attributed to a bodily function. As noted in chapter 3, the most dramatic case is that reported by Slawson and Davison (1964) in which a twenty-nine-year-old woman bit off the tip of her tongue. She attributed the blame to the tongue itself which, she explained, had an urge to be bitten. The urge was so strong and so unpleasant that she macerated the skin on her fingers and hands by continually using them to keep her teeth apart so that they could not bite her tongue. Interestingly the urge was much more unpleasant for her than the excruciating pain she felt immediately after biting her tongue. Before dismissing such behavior as totally bizarre we should remind ourselves of the urgency of the demand that continual itching creates for us to vigorously, and often painfully, scratch ourselves.

Self-scratching can be highly damaging as Allen and Harris (1966) note in their description of a five-year-old girl who scratched herself so much that her face and neck were literally covered with open sores from over a year of scratching. Allen and Harris view the self-scratching as a direct response (respondent behavior) to skin irritation. Most of us can recall moments when we have vigorously rubbed or even bitten body parts which were distressing us. The tongue biting of Slawson's mutilator may be a more dramatic and extreme form of similar body-engendered behavior.

Slawson's patient injured her hands in an attempt to control what she perceived as an offensive bodily part—her tongue. Other patients have taken a different tack; they have destroyed a part of their body which has been perceived as offensive. For example, Blacker and Wong (1962) described four male patients with strong feminine identification who repudiated their masculinity by removing their genitals, thus ridding themselves of "an offending organ." These patients had a history of more minor genital mutilation. For example, one patient at age six:

> Would place water between the prepuce and glans of the penis, then stick pins through the foreskin and watch the water come out. [P. 170]

In most instances the body location of the self-mutilating act probably has some personalized significance, whether actual or symbolic. In the foregoing instances, the acts were specifically directed to correct an aversive physical condition or to engender a preferred physical state. For example, Blacker and Wong (1962) talk of self-castrators as having a "vagina need." Some self-mutilation has been ascribed to autoeroticism, that is, the individual seeks sexual gratification through his body rather than through another person. Any part of the body, it is assumed, can be used for self-mutilation which is essentially masturbatory in purpose (Podvoll, 1969; Siomopoulos, 1974). Podvoll also notes that some mutilators attack their bodies to prevent them from indulging their narcissistic desires. They treat their bodies with "scorn and contempt" in order to control their love of their body. The idea that self-inflicted lacerations may be related to basic body narcissism is quite common (Gardner and Gardner, 1975; Kafka, 1969). Kafka, in his five-year psychoanalytic study of a self-cutting woman patient, suggests that she responded to her body in a way similar to the way in which children respond to their security blankets. She used her body as a "transitional object" which, when she cut it, gave her the security of knowing she was alive:

> As long as one has blood, one carried within oneself this potential security blanket capable of giving warmth and comforting envelopment. [P. 209]

The patient had fantasies "that an invisible layer around her stopped snowballs at some distance from her body." Kafka suggests that his patient viewed her body as a "not-me" object and as an object of fascination of an erotic kind.

The confusion of self and not-self is frequently reported and the body is described as a reference point to help the individual to distinguish the two. By cutting the body the individual highlights the distinction. In general, as Goldfarb (1958) notes, pain may help children to learn to distinguish between self and the world outside. Self-mutilation may serve an educational purpose.

A pet ploggle of investigators from all disciplines is menstruation. Authors not only draw an analogy between the bleeding of menstruation and the bleeding of self-mutilators, but also specifically suggest that self-cutting occurs at particular points of the menstrual cycle (Asch, 1971; Rosenthal et al., 1972). Self-cutting has even been referred to as "displaced genital bleeding" (Asch, 1971), and "vicarious menstruation" (Rosenthal et al., 1972). Rosenthal and his colleagues report that 65 percent of their cutters had a negative reaction to the menarche, whereas control subjects (noncutting suicide attempters) had been happy at the onset of menstruation. Moreover, the cutters had more irregular menstrual periods and more frequent amenorrhea than the controls. The evidence for a menstrual cycle/self-mutilation link is not strong, and it is somewhat difficult to generalize this explanation of self-mutilation to self-cutting in males.

Finally, we should note that head banging has been explained as a response to body conditions such as fatigue, (Collins, 1965; Gessell and Ilg, 1943) and middle-ear disease (DeLissovoy, 1962). However, a review of the evidence for the latter hypothesis was not supported (Carr, 1977). Whereas inner-ear disease may be found in some head bangers, it is an inadequate explanation for the majority of cases.

Head banging has also been discussed in terms of a pacemaking hypothesis which suggests that the banging represents the child's attempts to mimic its own heartbeat or to reexperience the mother's heartbeat which was felt in utero or while being held during infancy (Collins, 1965). However, this hypothesis has been rejected by studies such as that of DeLissovoy (1962) in which measurement of the tempo of the heartbeat has been found not to be correlated with head banging.

Conditioning

Standing in distinct contrast to the multitude of psychodynamic explanations of self-mutilation are those less colorful but more parsimonious explanations of this behavior which are based on behavior theory.

The majority of the behavioral accounts of self-mutilation adopt the position that self-mutilation is an operant response; a behavior which is acquired and maintained by the rewarding consequences it engenders. Among the obvious potential reinforcers for such behavior are the effects it has in terms of personal attention, solicitation, and bodily contact. It is very difficult for people not to respond to individuals who have mutilated themselves. Even if the observer's response is one of revulsion, it can be highly rewarding for the individual whose need for attention is continually or temporarily high—even negative attention can be better than no attention at all. In many instances the revulsion his audience displays, the distress his mutilation engenders, may be highly rewarding for the mutilator.

Isolation, medical treatment, lecturing, reprimands, surveillance, and many other apparently aversive consequences may represent to the mutilator important payoffs for his behavior and may maintain it at a high level of frequency. Even physical punishment may be highly rewarding to the mutilator since it involves stimulation, attention, and contact, which he may not be able to obtain by other means.

There is an abundance of observations, at least in the case of repetitive head banging or self-slapping behavior in institutionalized children, that support the view that self-mutilation is a function of its social consequences (Johnson, 1973;

Johnson, et al., 1975; Lucero et al., 1976; Morrison, 1972; Myers, 1975; Myers and Deibert, 1971; Offer and Barlow, 1960; Peterson and Peterson, 1968; Ragain and Anson, 1976; Repp and Deitz, 1974). It does, of course, make sense to most of us to think that the mutilator must be getting something out of his behavior. Believing this may even reassure us. More solid support for a behavioral account of such behavior comes from the evidence that experimentally altering the consequences of self-mutilating behavior directly affects the frequency of the behavior. Lovaas et al. (1965) have clearly demonstrated that self-injurious behavior can be greatly *increased* in rate when contingent social reinforcement is given.

It is possible that self-mutilating behavior in adolescents and adults represents an extension of behavior which was first learned in infancy (Green, 1967). Little evidence is available regarding the early history of self-mutilators, but it may be worthwhile to entertain the hypothesis that repetitive rocking and head banging in infants may represent responses by which sensory or socially deprived infants obtain stimulation. The remarkable persistence of these behaviors may be readily interpreted in terms of intermittent reinforcement or punishment conditions which make them resistant to extinction. The parents are likely to reinforce this behavior or punish it on an inconsistent schedule and to do so particularly when the responses are excessive. They thereby create ideal conditions for strengthening these behaviors and ensuring their persistence.

Individuals who have learned to head bang, scratch, pull their hair out, and so on, in infancy may attempt to respond to stressful situations encountered in later years by similar adaptations and to progress to more serious and dramatic forms which would have a higher probability of being reinforced in adolescence than would rocking or head banging.

A further explanation of self-mutilation in learning theory terms is based on an aversive conditioning model. Skinner's (1953) interpretation of masochism is helpful in this instance. He suggested that individuals might learn to behave in masochistic ways as a result of the following experiences.

1. Individuals might learn to expose themselves to aversive pain producing stimulation if by so doing they are able to avoid even more aversive consequences. Their self-injurious behavior may be an adaptive response which protects them from greater pain. Their self-mutilating behavior represents a "lesser evil." For example, prisoners have been reported to have mutilated themselves in order to be transferred to another cell-block and, thereby, avoid being forced to engage in homosexual activity. Soldiers have been known to injure themselves deliberately in order to avoid combat.

A child who has frequently been physically abused by his parents may learn to avoid further violence by injuring himself. The parent intent on abusing the child may decline to do so when he sees that the child is already abused (Green, 1968; Money, Wolff, and Annecillo, 1972).

2. Otherwise aversive or pain producing stimuli may acquire reinforcing properties by being paired with rewarding stimuli. Several laboratory studies with animals have demonstrated that animals can be trained to seek shock which normally would be highly aversive to them by involving them in training sessions in which shock was given on some trials in which their behavior led to reward in the form of food. By carefully presenting shock and food at the same time the shock, as it were, came to acquire reward value and the animal would subsequently emit the behavior even when food was not forthcoming and the only "reward" was pain.

Many studies have shown that otherwise aversive stimuli can come to function as stimuli which signal to the animal that a reward is forthcoming (and thus motivate the animal to respond). They may come to serve as actual rewards for behavior (Brown, Martin, and Morrow, 1964; Holz and Azrin, 1961; Murray and Nevin, 1967; Sandler, 1964). An example of a similar explanation of the acquisition of self-mutilating behavior in humans is that of a stimulus-deprived infant who learns to slap itself in order to obtain the stimulation of contact with the mother. To the observer who has not seen the early parent-child interaction, the head banging may appear painful, but to the child it may be associated with pleasure which may continue to motivate the child to slap itself long after the mother has ceased to respond. The behavior can become autonomous as pain comes to be perceived as pleasurable through simple conditioning.

Pigeons have been found to shock themselves hundreds of times just by giving them food now and again for doing so (Sandler, 1964). The analogy to self-mutilation in humans is apparent.

Self-esteem

A popular way of explaining self-mutilation is that it is a reaction to low self-esteem. Few investigators (present authors included) would quarrel with the findings of the many studies which have shown self-mutilators to have a poor self-image, feelings of worthlessness, or doubts about their ability to function adequately (Crabtree and Grossman, 1974; McKerracher, Loughane, and Watson, 1968; Mintz, 1964; Offer and Barlow, 1960). The low self-esteem may be related to a more general depression, may be a function of guilt or powerlessness, or be engendered by rejection, frustration, or even institutionalization. Of course, low self-esteem may be both a precursor and a consequence of self-mutilation.

However, as an explanation of self-mutilatory behavior, low self-esteem is somewhat unsatisfactory. For instance, self-mutilation has a low probability of occurrence in the many individuals who lack self-esteem. How can we differentiate between low self-esteem which engenders self-mutilation and low self-esteem which does not? Clearly, mutilating oneself is a dramatic act which is likely to gain an individual recognition and attention. The mutilator is likely to increase his chances of being "counted." He may well obtain status with his patient peers by his behavior. He may even be viewed as somewhat of a hero, a martyr. He is not likely to be unaware of the fact that even those who are most disgusted by his behavior still have some uncontrollable admiration for his bravery, his ability to withstand pain. He may even recognize that his act of self-mutilation may provide a few moments of excitement in the monotony of institutional life not only for himself and his peers but also for his staff. His self-injurious behavior may be therapeutic, in a way, for the staff. It can relieve their boredom. It can also make them feel they are really needed. It can reassure the staff member that he is different from his patients. In such ways self-mutilation can lead the patient with low self-esteem to feel important. But, in itself, it does not explain why the patient chooses self-mutilation. Given information about low self-esteem, we certainly cannot predict that self-mutilation will or will not occur.

Conclusions

The mind-boggling array of explanations offered for self-mutilating behavior not only reflect the host of disciplines which have studied this phenomenon but often represent the rigid loyalty of the investigator to a particular school of thought. There is a distinct lack of any coherent theory, even less an attempt to integrate the hodgepodge of conjecture, hypotheses, speculation, post hoc interpretation, suggestions, and commentaries. Further confusion is added to this bewildering scene when some authors choose to employ both different explanations and different levels of explanation for the same behavior. Correlations are proposed and presented without data. Data are presented without statistical test or interpretation. Very few of the hypotheses have been derived from theory, data or some form of functional analysis of the behavior. Rather than examine the behavior per se, many investigators choose to see it as symbolic or symptomatic of some underlying causative ploggly. Some plogglies are delightful but, unfortunately, their potential for translation into efficaceous prevention and control strategies remains problematic.

Almost all of the explanations imply deficiency either through some form of hereditary malfunction or through psychopathology. It is seen as perverse, beyond control, dysfunctional, and crazy behavior. A few writers allude to the pressures of the environment, the situational stresses, or the cultural framework of the act. Rarely do investigators ask why those with similar heredity, pressures, personality characteristics, early environments, creative urges, and institutional histories do *not* mutilate. Few, if any explanations lead to prediction; fewer still are parsimonious. Almost all are post hoc.

One reason for the shortcomings of explanations of self-mutilation is the almost insurmountable difficulties encountered in conducting research on self-mutilation in institutions. Many administrative officials in such settings are reluctant to acknowledge publicly that self-mutilation does in fact occur among patients in their jurisdiction. This sensitivity to publicity and possible adverse public opinion when attention is drawn to this problem presents the potential investigator with a variety of stumbling blocks. In the armamentarium of the reluctant administrator are oaths of secrecy prior to access to certain populations, requirements that proposals or reports be submitted to higher administrative officials for review, limiting access to the population, limiting access to confidential data, and red tape.

Our research milieu consisted of a progressive ministry , generous funding, concerned administrators, a responsive community, and a highly competent professional and support staff. Still, we encountered many of these obstacles. We can only speculate on the experience of investigators in less facilitative contexts.

There is much to criticize in our correctional and psychiatric institutions and a veritable legion of critics ready, willing, and able to accommodate. The administrators know full well that publicity is given mainly to the negative or sensational aspects of their services. For the protection of their institution and themselves they must quickly become astute politicians. They are, in the instance of self-mutilation, caught in a peculiar web of purpose. The administrator, it is reasoned, is entrusted with the care of an institutional population and hence responsible and accountable for the incidents which take place in his jurisdiction. The institutional administrator, then, must develop credible public explanations for the potentially sensational behaviors of those under his care. Self-mutilation is one such behavior. In many instances of dealing with critics, reference to a list of inadequacies is sufficient: inadequate funds, facilities, public support, and staff.

In some settings administrative practices are developed to cope with this problem. The "public face" denies or minimizes the problem. Patients may be required to wear clothing that covers evidence of their mutilation when in or near a public zone. When the public does intrude they may be provided with special tours which prevent them from being "exposed" to the mutilator. Subtle allusions to avoiding a "zoolike" atmosphere may be made by the guide to justify his reluctance to allow the visitor to see a mutilated patient. Procedural devices are formulated, such as moving a mutilator from ward to ward, transferring them to other service facilities, or even returning them expeditiously to the community—devices we dubbed *inmate checkers*.

In view of the impact of reports on self-mutilation, it is perhaps surprising that administrators are not more opposed to research. Convincing an administrator that the negative effects that might accrue from publication of a research project might be outweighed by its potential long-term benefits would prove a task of some magnitude.

Research on self-mutilation is not an attractive area for researchers. In many respects it has the status of a taboo topic. Moreover, the problems of achieving any approximation to methodological rigor are staggering, the ethical dilemmas are a veritable nightmare, and the tried-and-true laboratory-derived techniques of the social scientist are frequently unworkable in application. The notion of manipulating variables to produce observable effects has powerful consequences when the behavioral outcome is the mutilation of a body. The literature available to date must stand as testimony to the ingenuity, persistence, and perhaps even the perversity of these investigators.

5 Treatment of Self-Mutilation

During the years that we were attempting to treat the mutilating adolescents at Grandview we never ceased to be amazed by the response of visitors when they heard about the girls' carving and about our impressive inability to cope with it. Our innovative experimental treatment programs often (too often) attracted the attention of the social agencies around the province. Many hundreds of visitors came to have a look. Our adolescent offenders began to feel that they were living in a zoo. The visitors included many psychiatrists, psychologists, social workers, and other professionals in the mental health field. What amazed us was the ability of almost all of these visitors to tell us, after an afternoon's tour of the institution, precisely how we should treat the girls so as to eliminate self-mutilation. Each visitor had his own pet theory as to the most efficacious intervention strategy, environmental manipulation, recreational program, counseling or therapy technique that should be adopted. We were impressed by their confidence and optimism. The authoritative quality of their pronouncements often served to entrench the diminished self-esteem which had been engendered in us by the abject failure of our best treatment efforts. We had kept ourselves abreast of the literature in the field and had already tried many of the approaches that some of our visitors had recommended as "the" treatment. Our interns proposed with assurety that we should adopt their favorite approaches (ranging from Gestalt psychotherapy to firing the superintendent!). It did seem like such a very simple thing to dissuade someone from doing something to herself which was causing her harm.

At the risk of offending our reader, we would be willing to wager that having read the chapters describing the nature of self-mutilation and its possible explanation, you have already formed your own bias as to what we should have done with our clients at Grandview. It may well be that your treatment of choice is among those which have already been used with self-mutilators and which we will discuss in this chapter. Before we review the literature on the treatment of self-mutilation and before we describe the outcome of our treatment studies at Grandview, we ask you to take note of the views you have at the moment so that you might compare or contrast them with the views expressed in the literature and with those we adopted when we finally developed an effective way of treating the Grandview carvers. You may be reassured; more likely you will be surprised.

It was rather difficult to review the literature on the treatment of self-mutilation because investigators tend in their reports to give far more attention to describing the details of the mutilation, preferring to present ingenious explanations of the phenomenon rather than documenting how they tried to solve the problem.

It is often difficult to fathom what was actually done to treat the patient because the specifics of the treatment are seldom detailed in the reports. It is rare that one finds a program particularly geared to the treatment of self-mutilation itself. With some notable exceptions, therapists have attempted to treat self-mutilators with those well-established therapeutic modalities which have been judged to be valuable with a wide range of other problem behaviors. Although we have classified the material according to type of modality, we should note that a program will often be described within several sections. This is because in the treatment of self-mutilation many therapists adopt an eclectic approach.

Psychotherapy

With few exceptions, reports on psychotherapy with self-mutilating patients do not describe the treatment in any detail. They focus on a description of the patient, his or her self-mutilatory behavior, and the psychodynamics underlying the symptoms. Surprisingly, the results of the treatment effort are seldom even mentioned and the reader is left only to presume that therapy was successful. Most of the material is anecdotal, drawn from case history data. Few programs include follow-up. Needless to say, controlled experiments are rendered problematic in this field because clinicians are reluctant to withhold a potentially promising treatment for control group comparison.

Partial justification for a psychotherapy approach can be found in the research of Nelson and Grunebaum (1971), Shodell and Reiter (1968), and Simpson (1975), who have provided evidence of the relationship between difficulty in verbalizing emotions and self-mutilatory behavior. Simpson (1975) has noted that cutters experience substantial difficulty in verbalizing their needs, making traditional psychotherapy difficult. Reviewing the cases of twenty-four wrist cutters, in fourteen cases improved verbal facility was associated with clinical improvement and cessation of cutting after brief, extensive psychotherapy. Shodell and Reiter (1968) reported that verbal schizophrenic children were significantly less likely to mutilate than nonverbal schizophrenic children. They argue that the ability to verbalize in schizophrenic children would enable them to use language as a substitute for action when releasing their tension and frustration.

In a study of wrist slashers who had cut their wrists five to six years previously, Nelson and Grunebaum (1971) found that more than half were well or substantially improved. Patient improvement was attributed to: (1) increased ability to verbalize feelings, (2) use of constructive action at times of emotional crisis, and (3) control of psychotic delusions through psychiatric follow-up and medication. The authors go on to suggest:

> The optimal treatment of the wrist slasher involves an alliance between patient and doctor and the reinforcement of patients' ego controls over their symptoms through an approach that combines education, identification with the therapist, and an appropriate mixture of permissiveness and limit setting. [P. 1349]

Siomopoulos (1974) has described the success of several cases in which psychotherapy was focused on the presumed sexual dynamics of the patient's behavior. One case was a twenty-seven-year-old single woman who had been admitted to the hospital after repeated self-cutting and scratching on her arms, breasts, and abdomen. Her self-cutting followed intense feelings of mounting tension. "She continued cutting herself almost daily until . . . the therapist began exploring with her the relationship between her cuttings and her attitudes towards sex, masturbation, and her early upbringing (p.88). The described cases were of female self-cutters whose persistent cutting stopped when the therapist began discussing their early upbringing and their attitudes toward sex and masturbation.

Novotny (1972) reported success in the use of a variety of treatments with a diverse group of self-mutilating patients. With some patients an interpretation of dependency needs and wishes for attention was helpful. With others, an interpretation of the anger and hostility seemed to help to control this particular kind of behavior. Unfortunately, no data are presented by which one can evaluate success with these patients.

One of the more detailed accounts of a psychotherapeutic encounter with a self-mutilating patient has been provided by Crabtree (1967). The patient, Jane, had "attempted to break windows; she set fires at various places, she attacked another patient; she eloped from the hospital; she took an overdose of aspirin . . .; she swallowed a needle" (p. 93). Although prior psychotherapeutic intervention had failed with this patient, Crabtree reports the cessation of self-mutilatory behavior after the first year of intensive psychotherapy, the early goal of which "should be the translation of this form of mutilation into an object-oriented dilemma by the establishment and maintenance of an interactional, transference psychosis, for which a way out can be sought" (p. 91).

Reports of the treatment of self-mutilation often mention, without elaboration, that psychotherapy has been used as one technique in a multimodal approach to treatment (for example, Blacker and Wong, 1962; Matthews, 1968; Merbaum, 1973). In other cases the elaboration is interesting. For example, Stinnett and Hollender (1970) report on a case of compulsive eye banging. The young male patient had been hospitalized several times and had been treated unsuccessfully by psychotherapy, chemotherapy, and aversive stimulation. One program of psychotherapy enabled him to resist the impulse to hit himself, although he still reported an urge to do so. "He [the patient] believed that therapy was helpful, not because of the insight he had gained, but because the therapist was so nice to him—treated him more like a friend than a patient" (p. 372). A second course of psychotherapy some eight years later was instituted after the patient had struck himself to the point of detaching the retina of one eye. In the hospital after surgery his arms had been placed in casts to prevent further injury. Psychotherapy enabled the patient to resist hitting his eyes although he continued to touch and press his eyeballs. Six months later he was readmitted and placed in restraints. He had again succeeded in detaching the retina of the same eye. This time corrective surgery was unsuccessful. However, it was reported that some control of his impulse was established. The patient was discharged and formed a supportive relationship with a rabbi. In summarizing the case of this patient, the authors conclude that where a patient's ego is strong enough to contain the impulse, interpretative psychotherapy is possible. (Not true in this case.) As emergency measures they suggest that the therapist "focus . . . primarily on bolstering the ego instead of reducing the force of the impulse. Unfortunately, measures such as medications and conditioning are of little benefit. Only the magically imbued power of a therapist or a clergyman is likely to accomplish the task of reinforcing the controlling mechanisms. When these, too, prove inadequate, physical restraint is required" (p. 374).

Where eclectic programs have appeared to show promise it is regrettable that research methodology is lacking which would enable one to reach firm conclusions as to the efficacy of particular components. For instance, Hawkins, Jones, and Tibbetts (1956) report on ten patients referred to a hospital for psychiatric assessment after incidents of deliberate self-injury. All ten were involved in psychotherapy, and six of these were also treated by narcoanalysis. Hawkins and co-workers report that half of the ten patients made satisfactory progress.

A major decrease in the self-mutilatory behavior of hospitalized adolescent psychiatric patients was achieved in a program described by Crabtree and Grossman (1974). They attributed their success to a number of factors: the establishment of a "wholesome community," an "atmosphere of trust and good-feeling," the introduction of "administrative clarity," and an "open door" policy. They also noted that patients and staff were persuaded to "work more closely with high-risk patients." Presumably, the combination of these factors led to the 94 percent decrease in self-mutilation which Crabtree and Grossman reported. This result is the most, if not the only, dramatically successful outcome described in the literature, and it is regrettable that the program did not provide experimental controls which would enable us to conclude that the improvement was not attributable to Hawthorne effects or simply to the passage of time. Moreover, Crabtree and Grossman do not describe their program in sufficient detail to allow us to evaluate the importance of particular aspects of their complex program or to enable other therapists to replicate their work. This program is clearly important to the development of successful intervention techniques for self-mutilation, and we hope it will be investigated further in more controlled trials.

There are few reports of group psychotherapy with self-mutilators. Roback et al. (1972) utilized group psychotherapy in a multifaceted treatment approach designed for a patient who had cut and burned her arms and face. Although a prior group psychotherapy experience had been unsuccessful another attempt was undertaken. The patient was involved in weekly sessions "which stressed interpersonal interaction and 'crisis intervention.' The therapists in the group attempted to model spontaneity for the patient and socially reinforced all positive social responses she performed" (p. 191). The authors report that her mutilative behavior was eliminated and improvement maintained during a four-month follow-up period.

Offer and Barlow (1960) describe and analyze a series of incidents of self-mutilation by a group of twelve young patients. Over a nine-month period ninety incidents occurred of which 90 percent were attributed to these patients. Group psychotherapy sessions were held "which helped decrease the number of incidents to their 'usual' prevalence" (p. 194).

Frequently, clininicans, in describing their work with self-mutilators, note that prior to their intervention their patients had been unsuccessfully treated by psychotherapy. There appear to be as many reports of the failure of psychotherapy as there are of its success.

Some self-injurious behaviors are remarkably resistant to treatment. For example, Slawson and Davidson (1964) studied a twenty-nine-year-old hysterical woman who repeatedly mutilated her tongue by biting. A three-month program of psychotherapy temporarily reduced her self-mutilatory behavior, but later the symptom reappeared. Slawson and Davidson state: "She continues as an out-patient, but she has been unable to work and is totally dependent on her family. The psychotherapeutic approach has been warm, kindly, and supportive" (p. 584). Slawson and Davidson reported that they also tried sodium amytal, chlopromazine, hypnosis, "anaclitic therapy," "educative therapy," behavioral conditioning, and electroconvulsive therapy. No program was successful.

Morgan, Barton, and Pottle (1976) reported a study of 279 patients who were followed up one to two years after an act of nonfatal, deliberate self-harm. Those who received more prolonged psychiatric care immediately after self-harm were significantly more likely than others to show repetition in the following twelve months. If self-harm is associated with a degree of secondary gain, intervention aimed at relieving distress and providing social help after self-harm may increase the likelihood that such behavior will be repeated.

We should note that many investigators have suggested that self-mutilating patients often deliberately and explicitly reject attempts to involve them in psychotherapy or at attempts by family physicians, clergy, or friends to lend a sympathetic ear.

Psychotherapy has potential for harm as well as health. Miller and Bashkin (1974), for example, have described self-mutilation which occurred in a young man who injured himself in response to impending separation from his therapist. Pao (1969) has also described how self-mutilation may be triggered by the patient's feelings of abandonment and has suggested that such issues should be discussed early in treatment even at the risk of precipitating self-injurious behavior. Burnham (1969) has noted that therapists may respond to their patient's behavior with guilt or anger and increased efforts to protect the patient from herself–efforts which may lead to increased tension and guilt in the patient and a concomitant increase in self-mutilation.

Chemotherapy

Drug treatment in the control of self-destructive behavior has been widely used. However, the evidence for its efficacy is more difficult to find. Only one experimental study (Varga and Simpson, 1971) provided a controlled evaluation of the effect of drug administration on self-mutilatory behavior. Loxapine was administered to sixteen chronically institutionalized male patients who required physical restraints to prevent self-injury or who posed extremely difficult management problems. Neither ward, staff, nor patients were aware of the nature of the drug, and placebo was used during baseline assessment. Each patient's clinical status was rated on global measures, and physical changes were evaluated through laboratory tests (blood and urine samples, heart rate, blood pressure). Of the ten patients who completed the study (several were dropped due to adverse side effects such as seizures), three showed no change and seven were rated as minimally improved. The greatest general improvement was shown by three schizophrenic patients. Varga and Simpson concluded that "uncontrollable self-destructive behavior was not notably benefited in this study."

The few positive results reported for chemotherapy are largely anecdotal reports of one patient. The treatment effect is often confounded by the concurrent administration of another therapy. For example, Cooper and Fowlie (1973) report "satisfactory control with lithium carbonate of gross self-mutilation in a severely subnormal girl in her early twenties" (p. 370). Her behavior consisted of gnawing at the back of her hands until they were ulcerated. It is reported that her mutilatory behavior did not reappear in a five-year follow-up.

Two of four cases of autocastration noted by Blacker and Wong (1963) were administered trifluoperazine, and all four were reported to be functioning well after varying lengths of follow-up. One patient was responding well to chlorpromazine. In each case medication was given after the patient had castrated himself. On the other hand, Tanner and Zeiler (1975) reported that doses of chlorpromazine and trifluoperazine had no effect on a patient's self-slapping but did increase the amount of time she spent sleeping.

Peterson and Peterson (1968), in a discussion of the severe self-destructive behaviors of an eight-year-old boy, reported that their subject received thioridazine and chlorpromazine prior to and during most of their study. Having noted the period during which drugs were not administered, they concluded that no relationship appeared between the presence and absence of medication and the rate of self-destructive behavior.

Slawson and Davidson (1964) prescribed chemotherapy for their hysterical patient who severely and repeatedly bit her own tongue. On one of several hospital admissions she is described as "severely depressed to the point of stupor." She remained depressed for three months, but after treatment with psychotherapy and phenothiazines she was discharged as "notably improved" (p. 582). The patient did relapse, however, and during this hospitalization, amytal interviews were started with some temporary improvement. Following a severe tongue bite, chlorpromazine was adminstered and controlled her general hyperactivity. At another treatment stage, trifluoperazine was successful in controlling severe agitation. "There has been no other improvement" (p. 585).

Asch (1971), in a report on wrist scratching among girls, suggested that their self-mutilatory behavior was stimulation seeking. As a preventative measure he suggested that small doses of amphetamines for a few days might be helpful in countering their anhedonic feelings (emptiness, deadness). However, no cases were reported.

A patient successfully treated for self-cutting and burning in a multifactorial program was administered parnate and haloperidol for symptomatic relief of "anhedonic feeling and poor impulse control" (Roback et al., 1972, p. 190). Because of the many treatment methods employed, efficacy of drug administration effects cannot be assessed.

Some decrease in the self-injurious behavior of a retarded, adolescent head banger treated by Haldol during a behavior modification program was observed by Martin and Treffry (1970). Previous attempts at drug therapy (unsuccessful) had included large doses of anticonvulsive drugs, tranquilizers, and sedatives whenever staff requested them because of the boy's extreme noisiness and abusiveness.

Another unsuccessful case of chemotherapy is reported by Simpson (1973). A patient who repeatedly mutilated her genitalia was first treated by antidepressants and electroconvulsive shock and then by narcotherapy. The patient's self-mutilation was "associated with episodes of anorexia, . . . and a wide range of acting-out behavior" (p. 808).

In describing the treatment history of a self-injuring child, Muttar et al. (1975) reported that their patient, at the age of six, had been hospitalized and discharged on chlorpromazine. On readmission for her continuing self-destructive behavior, chlorpromazine, trichloryl, diazepam, nitrazepam, haloperidol,

L-dopa, and E panutin were administered and "ineffective except in hypnotic doses" (p. 5).

Negative reports of the outcome of drug treatments are made for a variety of drugs and patient types. Miller and Bashkin (1974) found that high doses of phenothiazines were ineffective in controlling the self-mutilatory behavior of a patient described as "in a state of extreme confusion, perplexity, disorientation [with] marked psychomotor retardation . . . His behavior was characterized by indifference, negativism, and mutism" (p. 639).

As an illustration of the difficulties encountered in treating head banging of severely retarded adults, Collins (1964) discovered that "ataractic drugs, in dosages high enough to produce toxic side effects, produced only slight and temporary improvement" (p. 207).

Unspecified drugs have also been reported as unsuccessful (Bryson et al., 1971; Crabtree, 1967; Saposnek and Watson, 1974).

Finally Tate (1972) has observed that "little evidence exists that drugs are beneficial with chronic self-mutilation except . . . at dosage levels which render the child vegetable like" (p. 72).

Electroconvulsive therapy

Electroconvulsive therapy (ECT) as a treatment for self-destructive behavior has usually been considered for the hospitalized adult only after the failure of both drug programs and psychotherapy. The results, as suggested by case history materials, are far from promising.

Brief periods of improvement, where they occurred at all, were typically followed by deterioration and renewed episodes of self-mutilation.

Temporary cessation of self-mutilation was reported by Blacker and Wong (1963) who employed ECT in a case of repeated genital self-mutilation. After a course of twelve treatments which was followed by a remission, he returned to work. At this stage, "he dropped therapy, became unable to function and was hospitalized for a month . . . After a brief course of ECT he returned to work" (p. 171). A relapse of self-mutilation ensued after one year. Cox and Klinge (1976) have also described temporary beneficial effects of ECT in a girl who exhibited a variety of self-mutilatory behaviors. She was readmitted ten months after treatment.

Miller and Bashkin (1974) described a wrist cutter who received ECT following an unsuccessful chemotherapy regimen:

> Thirteen electroconvulsant treatments were given, after which he slowly improved. He remained in the institution for another year, during which time he inflicted superficial lacerations on his forearms and wrists." [P. 639]

As time went on, his mutilative behavior became incessant and severe.

Bryson et al., (1971) reported the failure of numerous ECT treatments in cases of de Lange syndrome. A similar unsuccessful outcome was reported by Davidson (1962) for a patient who had self-enucleated an eye during an hallucia-tory episode:

> Electroconvulsive treatment and a full course of insulin comas did not improve his state . . . he then began to manifest self-mutilatory behavior of diverse kinds" [P. 290]

These behaviors included sawing his neck on a barbed wire fence (Davidson, 1962).

Failures to provide other than very temporary effects have been reported by Hawkins, Jones, and Tibbetts (1956), Roback et al. (1972) and Simpson (1973). Finally, Slawson and Davidson (1964) report the case of a twenty-nine-year-old woman who repeatedly mutilated her tongue by biting. Innumerable therapies and treatments were attempted with no success:

> It was with mixed feelings (on the part of the staff) that electroconvul-sive therapy was begun. The patient initially regarded it as the divine panacea. After six treatments there was no change in her condition. [P. 594]

Psychosurgery

The reader must by now have an appreciation of the intractability of self-mutila-ting behavior to the spectrum of traditional treatment methods. A few cases have been reported in which, as a final desperate measure, psychosurgery was performed.

In a symposium on self-mutilation, Burnham (1969) referred to a patient who had been hospitalized for some time as a "celebrated cutter and swallower." The patient:

> Finally provoked a prefrontal lobotomy. I have heard that this ended her cutting days, and that she afterward busied herself cutting paper dolls. [P. 224]

Balduzzi (cited in Stinnett and Hollender, 1970) reported that a fifty-year-old woman had destroyed her left eye by repetitively touching and pressing it while looking in a mirror. Her compulsion was apparently relieved by a trans-orbital leucotomy.

The most complete description of procedures and outcome is provided by Davidson's (1962) report on the treatment of a young man who eventually enucleated his own eye. An "open bilateral parafrontal leucotomy with bilateral section of the arterior thalamic radiation" was performed after all other treatments had failed (psychotherapy, chemotherapy, electroconvulsive shock). Interestingly, Davidson reported that when informed of the impending operation the patient became quiet and cooperative and ceased completely his attempts at self-mutilation (p. 291).

The post operative course is also described. The patient was first apathetic and then with remision of all psychotic symptoms became uninhibited, euphoric, and socially active. After discharge, schizoid personality traits reasserted themselves and one brief psychotic episode with slight self-mutilatory tendencies is reported. Davidson notes that in spite of some thought disturbance, he is able to work, live in an aftercare hostel, and take part in social activities.

Attention/Stimulation

For most people, the immediate response to the injury of another, and particularly the sight of blood, is attending: looking intensely, and making remarks that reflect concern, shock, sometimes horror. This is no less true if the wound is self-inflicted. Paying attention, showing concern, and the like, in addition to being the most probable initial response to a self-inflicted injury, have been used as core elements in attempts to treat the mutilator, to get him or her to stop.

The group of practitioners that has used attention, warmth, and support as a treatment for self-injuring has been supportive of the person and attentive to the wounds. In a review of cases selected from special schools and hospitals, Sandow (1975) found that giving attention and coaxing were the treatment methods most often reported by staff. While specific outcome data are not reported for this approach generally, it has not been effective in reducing self-injurious behavior. In fact, it has been suggested that giving attention is most likely to perpetuate the behavior (Bucher and Lovaas, 1968).

Collins (1964) reported a case study of a severly retarded young man who had begun head banging in early childhood. The behavior had increased to the point that constant restraints were required. He was confined to bed with his limbs strapped down, a sheet restraining his trunk, and a thick foam rubber collar around his neck. The treatment program provided him with attention and stimulation throughout most of his waking hours. He was given a radio and squeaking squeeze toys. Mobiles were placed over his bed. He was given candy and gum at frequent intervals and perfumed soaps and lotions were used to bathe him. He was taken to the toilet eight times a day and two attendants spent fifteen minutes a day with him while restraints were removed. They took him on walks, played with him, and provided much physical contact. Within weeks the patient's efforts to head bang had subsided, and he was able to have longer periods out of restraints. Within a year he no longer required restraints. Collins suggested that the treatment program provided the opportunity for external stimulation and freedom of movement which enabled the patient to begin to reestablish his concept of body image through motor activity.

Along similar lines, some investigators have observed a reduction in the stereotyped movements frequently associated with self-injurious behavior in institutionalized population when normal outlets for activities and interests were provided (Berkson and Davenport, 1964; Green, 1967; Levy, 1944).

One facet of a treatment research program reported by Lovaas and Simmons (1969) included attention as a variable. To determine what factors in the environment were controlling the self-injurious behaviors of a young patient, the effects of three conditions were observed. First, the child was restrained in bed and given only routine care for twenty-four hours. No change in the rate of self-injury was observed. The same lack of effect was noted for continual attention, that is, social satiation. Attention given contingent on self-injurious behavior, however, markedly increased the rate. Lovaas and Simmons concluded that "in this instance the expression of 'love' contingent upon self-destructive behavior benefits only the giver" (p. 155).

Another case reported by Lovaas et al. (1965) supports this finding. The comment, "I don't think you're bad," made following self-injurious behavior by a young girl, greatly increased the rate of head banging and self-slapping.

Nonattending/Extinction

A more common treatment strategy for self-injurious behavior is the withholding of attention. Behavioral explanations suggest that self-mutilation is maintained by the attention it engenders. The individual learns that by mutilating he can obtain a considerable amount of attention from people which might not otherwise be forthcoming. Rather than increasing the staff's attention to the behavior the behavioral therapists urge withholding attention so that the behavior is not reinforced. According to the learning paradigm, the behavior under such circumstances is likely to be extinguished.

Some success has been reported with the use of behavior therapies for the treatment of self-injurious or destructive behavior. The target group has generally been children, often retarded or autistic, nearly always institutionalized. The behaviors treated have included head and back banging, self-scratching, biting, breaking windows with their head, pounding various parts of the body with fists, hands, knees, or against furniture or walls. Many of these children had been kept constantly in restraints to prevent permanent physical damage.

The basic premise of these approaches is that the self-destructive behavior is learned or instrumental and maintained by the child's environment. The emotional impact of self-destructive behavior on the observer has already been noted, as have the powerful responses they elicit from others (Ferster, 1968; Ross, 1977).

Gardner (1965) treated a child's psychosomatic seizures and associated tantrums with these procedures in a family context. The child's parents were trained to ignore the seizure and tantrum behaviors and to attend only to appropriate behavior. The study included reversal and reinstatement periods, and a follow-up after one year showed no recurrence of the target behaviors.

Bucher and Lovaas (1968) extinguished the head banging of a seven-year-old retardate who had previously been in restraints. He was released from restraints for half an hour a day for eight days while in his bed. During these periods no attention was paid to his self-injurious behaviors. At the end of this period, he no longer hit his head while unrestrained. There was no change in his rate of self-injurious behavior in other situations. The authors also report that the child banged his head more than *ten thousand times* during the extinction procedure!

Duker (1975) presents an interesting analysis of the self-destructive behavior of a young Lesch-Nyhan syndrome patient after thirteen two-and-one-half-hour sessions of having the staff ignore self-destructive responses and encourage adaptive behavior. Self-biting and associated crying and whining were virtually eliminated. Unfortunately, it was not possible to follow the same procedure for head banging, due to the danger of permanent injury, and the child had to be restrained in a chair.

A twenty-four-week program of social isolation with two-hour sessions twice a day was successful in eliminating multiple self-injurious behaviors in a nine-year-old autistic child (Jones, Simmons, and Frankel, 1974). Major improvement was found, and it was possible to terminate the social isolation sessions. The behavior later reappeared and was again dramatically reduced by reinstatement of the program.

Martin and Treffry (1970) engineered an environment for a severely retarded girl who had been face slapping and head banging to the point of requiring physical restraint. The girl, who refused to walk, was placed on a chair behind a cardboard screen to ensure that she would not receive any form of reinforcement for her self-injurious behavior. The screen also served to provide clear cues to the staff to prevent inadvertent reinforcement of the target behavior. Care was taken to structure all contact with the patient. At mealtime food was placed nearby; she was instructed to eat and left alone for a set period of time after which her tray was removed. The patient was reinforced at frequent intervals following minimal periods of self-injury. Martin and Treffry reported that the application of this type of treatment regimen resulted in a decrease of the self-injurious behavior, enabling them to develop a program to increase her mobility and self-care skills.

Additional discussion of the value of extinction precedures as a controlling device for self-injurious behavior are presented by Carr (1977) and Lester (1972). The practictioner who wishes to use extinction techniques must recognize their shortcomings and dangers. It is in the nature of the extinction process that initially the response will occur with greater frequency before it is gradually eliminated. This poses an obvious problem for the use of extinction as a treatment for self-injurious behaviors and may put the client in physical jeopardy when the behavior is severe (Bucher and Lovaas, 1968; Ducker, 1975).

Many staff members are simply unable to refrain from attending to the self-mutilating patient, thus rendering extinction procedures impossible (Bachman, 1972; Sandow, 1975). Moreover, in institutional settings it is difficult to ensure that all staff members refrain from attending to the self-injurious behavior. This failure can create conditions of intermittent reinforcement which will increase the persistence of the behavior. The same condition may result from accidental reinforcement, which too often occurs when many staff members are involved with the patient.

Extinction, when it is successful, is a very gradual process. The mutilator must learn through experience that his behavior does not pay off. Typically many trials are required in which the patient injures himelf in the absence of reinforcement. In some instances several hundred pairings of the behavior and nonreinforcement are required before extinction is completed. In the case of self-mutilating acts, an extinction procedure might lead to termination of the behavior through extinction of the patient!

Time Out

Some investigators have employed a procedure known as *time out* from reinforcement. In this technique all social reinforcement for the behavior is removed for a specified period following a self-injury episode. Usually the patient is taken to an empty room or an isolated area contingent on the occurrence of the self-injurious behavior.

As with extinction, the use of time out may present physical danger to a severely self-harming patient left unrestrained. Tate and Baroff (1966) were forced to abandon the method for this reason, although they had found it had led to some reduction in head banging and self-slapping of a nine-year-old psychotic boy. Their time out had involved removal of physical contact contingent on self-injurious behavior.

Muttar et al. (1975) reported the failure of a contingent time out program in the treatment of a young girl who severely and persistently injured her eyes. After four weeks the program was discontinued as the patient expanded her self-injurious responses: she changed from fist to face banging, began head banging against hard objects, lost weight, and had to be medically treated daily for self-inflicted injuries. The patient was finally rendered stuporous by the administration of chlorpromazine.

To avoid this problem, some treatments have also included restraint during the time out period (Hamilton, Stephens, and Allen, 1967). These authors also observed the substitution of another form of self-injury on the elimination of the original response (in one case, the substitution of head and back banging for breaking windows with the head). Although these substitute behaviors were eventually eliminated by time out as well, they suggest the method may be most useful for treatment of single, invariable behaviors, that is, where the response is not too complex. Duker (1975) has suggested that time out by social isolation is the appropriate treatment choice for self-injurious behavior with a low magnitude and rate.

Wolf, Risley, and Mees (1964) reported, however, the elimination of tantrum and other self-injurious responses of a three-and-a-half-year-old child by employing contingent time out (he was sent to his room for thirty minutes) and reinforcement of positive behaviors. When the behavior recurred two years later in a nursery school setting, reinstatement of the procedure eliminated the tantrums in three time outs (removal from classroom).

The most serious drawback of this treatment method is succinctly summarized by Jones, Simmons and Frankel, (1974). They suggest that the staff, while struggling to remove a patient for a time out contingent on self-injurious behavior, may be inadvertently reinforcing the behavior they wish to eliminate. We would also note that it may be that a brief period of intense, self-engendered attention is much more reinforcing than the structured social reinforcements which are characteristic of programmed institutional environments.

Training Alternative Behaviors

Peterson and Peterson (1968) have suggested that therapists systematically train self-mutilators in alternative behaviors. They reason that many patients have few alternative responses in their repertoire or that they occur infrequently because they have been reinforced insufficiently. Although there are several variants of this procedure, it essentially involves attending to and reinforcing appropriate desired behavior and generally ignoring the self-injurious behavior. It does require that the patient be free from restraints so that alternative behaviors will occur. With extremely high rate self-injurious acts, few appropriate alternative behaviors may be available to reinforce (Lovaas et al., 1965).

Allen and Harris (1966) used this procedure to eliminate severe self-scratching of a young girl, using the child's mother as therapist. Under their supervision the other was taught to ignore the scratching and to reward other appropriate behaviors including not scratching. In addition to social reinforcements, tokens to be traded for toys were also dispensed. These extrinsic reinforcements were gradually withdrawn after six weeks. A four-month follow-up showed no recurrence of the behavior.

Ragain and Anson (1976) reported a demonstration of stimulus control of a retarded adolescent's head banging. Food, during the evening meal, was made contingent on a specified period free from self-injury (first fifteen seconds, then gradually increased to thirty seconds). On this differential reinforcement of other behavior (DRO) schedule, the subject's head banging was eliminated. The use of a noncontingent schedule produced an increase in the behavior which was reduced again by two further sessions of DRO. An interesting part of the study was Ragain and Anson's report that, after extinction, when the contingent reinforcement schedule was reinstituted "the girl was removed from the training room on three different occasions in order to stop tantrum behavior." Although the problem behaviors were not completely eliminated, it was demonstrated that stimulus control over self-mutilating behaviors can be achieved with this technique.

Lovaas et al. (1965) reinforced socially appropriate behavior of a nine-year-old hospitalized schizophrenic patient who banged and slapped her head. Social approval was found to be reinforcing. Rates of self-injurious behavior were recorded during the reinforcement of behavior that is appropriate to music, for example, singing and clapping. The appropriate behaviors were incompatible with her self-injurious responses. The occurrence and magnitude of self-injurious behavior varied directly with reinforcement of the incompatible behavior. When reinforcement was withheld (extinction), the rate of self-injurious behavior increased again. Interestingly, a later presentation of the songs used earlier during the reinforcement of clapping and singing reduced the rate of self-injurious behavior.

In contrast, Peterson and Peterson (1968) reinforced alternate, although not incompatible, behavior in their treatment of an eight-year-old hospitalized boy who would bang his head, cry, scream, and slap when a small blanket was removed. Food was used as a reinforcer, and time out was employed during the first phase of the study. In the second phase, the time out was eliminated, and the boy was instructed to walk across the room to a chair when he self-injured. This was continued until he walked from one chair to the other with no self-injury. After the second phase, the rate of self-injury was near zero.

Weiher and Harman (1975) reported on the use of omission training (OM) in eliminating head banging of a fourteen year old severely retarded boy. OM is described by the authors as "a response elimination technique which specifies reinforcement whenever a specified response is not emitted for a designated time." This strategy provides for rapid control over self-injurious behavior and the increase of alternative appropriate behavior which can then be positively reinforced by the staff members. The successful application of this technique enabled these investigators to institute further training for the patient free from physical restraints.

Time out and DRO have been combined in treatment programs with some positive results. For example, Brawley et al. (1968) used withdrawal of contact for 15 seconds following self-injury as time out, and social and food reinforcements for appropriate behavior such as verbalization, use of materials, and following requests. Control of this autistic child's severe self-slapping and tantrum behavior was demonstrated sequentially by baseline, reinforcement, reversal, and reinforcement phases. Three months after termination of treatment Brawley et al. reported that inappropriate behavior remained at a low level.

Duker (1975) used confinement to a small bathroom for ten minutes as time out and intermittent reinforcement of incompatible noninjurious behavior by attention and toys to reduce the head banging of a retarded adolescent to near zero. A previous program which required him to wear a helmet for half an hour after banging and positive reinforcement of positive behavior had been unsuccessful.

In an initial attempt to eliminated self-injurious behavior in two adolescents by 45-second withdrawal of attention and candy reinforcement for 15 seconds of no self-injury was unsuccessful (Corte, Wolff, and Locke, 1971). Changing the reinforcer to malt and conducting treatment at mealtimes (therefore creating mild deprivation) resulted in significant reduction in self-injury for both patients.

The use of combined methods in many studies precludes evaluation of the efficacy of a single treatment modality. Myers (1975) reported the comparison of three strategies in the treatment of a twelve-year-old retardate with a four-year history of finger and nail biting. Scolding, isolation from reinforcement, and taping his fingers had all been ineffective. Myers reported that extinction (twenty-four days of ignoring the behavior) had no effect. The use of token reinforcements for common compliance behavior (withheld during biting) stabilized and reduced the behavior, but at an unacceptably high level. Introducing response cost, taking away a token with verbal reprimand for biting, eliminated the behavior within twenty days. During this procedure, the subject continued to earn tokens for positive behavior and to trade them for toys and treats. After twelve weeks, there had been no recurrence of biting and no disruption of functioning in other areas. Myers pointed out that this subject was accustomed to a token economy as part of the training school program and did not engage in biting continuously.

Bachman (1972) has pointed out that the alternative behavior need not be incompatible with the self-injurious behavior (SIB). Rather,

> Just the fact of providing S with an alternative response that was efficient in producing positive reinforcement produced the subsequent decrease in SIB. [P. 215]

Bachman also notes that there are many practical difficulties in attempts to train alternative behaviors for patients in understaffed crowded settngs:

> The failure of the ward environment to reinforce alternative incompatible behaviors may have created, maintained and increased the self-injurious behavior in the first place. [P. 215]

Moreover, Duker (1975) has observed that patients test this approach by emitting alternative injurious behaviors (elbow hitting, vomiting, and self-biting). These behaviors tend, however, to diminish in frequency as training progresses.

Wolf, Risley, and Mees (1964) pointed out that a high frequency of self-injurious behavior may preclude the use of alternative behavior training.

Sandow (1975) has pointed out other difficulties in the application of behavioral techniques: the staff's limited understanding or inadequate application of the principles of behavior modification, institutional pressures which produce inconsistent reinforcement of alternative behaviors, and the high probability that the child will obtain secondary reinforcement from self-mutilatory behavior. Too often it is not possible to control the behavior of other professional groups or parents whose treatment of the child interferes with the reinforcement regimen, which must be followed consistently if the behavioral strategy is to be successful.

Punishment/Aversive Conditioning

The literature on self-mutilation is replete with reports of the successful treatment of self-injurious behavior by the application of contingent punishment. Electric shock, for example, delivered immediately following a self-injurious behavior has successfully reduced the rate to zero or near zero after a few applications (Ball et al., 1975; Bucher and Lovaas, 1968; Corte, Wolff, and Locke, 1971; Lovaas and Simmons, 1969; Merbaum, 1973; Muttar et al., 1975; Tate and Baroff, 1966; Wilbur, Chandler and Carpenter, 1974; and Wright, 1973). Detailed reviews of this literature have been presented by Bachman (1972), Carr (1977), Frankel and Simmons (1976), and Lester (1972).

Success with punishment other than shock has also been reported. Roback et al. (1972), for example, have described the success of their program with a self-burning patient which included withdrawal of privileges for twenty-four hours, contingent on occurrence of burning. Morrison (1972) nearly eliminated the severe head banging of a retarded child using a light tap on the head along with the verbal instruction, no. As is frequently the case in aversive conditioning programs, Morrison also provided concurrently reinforcement of other appropriate behaviors. Slawson and Davidson (1964) reported that a program of verbal reprimands (and praise for positive behaviors) for tongue biting was somewhat helpful in their treatment of a young woman. Aromatic ammonia contingent on self-slapping eliminated this behavior in an autistic woman (Tanner and Zeiler, 1975). Two cases are reported by Singh (1976) in which tapping fingers with a stick eliminated eye poking, and head banging was punished by the statement, "Don't do that." In both cases time out and DRO procedures with food were used concurrently at mealtimes.

A chronic schizophrenic patient who persisted in lacerating her arms was successfully treated by Berman (1975) using behavioral contracting. The patient's purse was taken away if new wounds appeared. Only two experiences with purse withdrawal as a punishment were required before the patient ceased self-mutilation. No further incidents of cutting occurred in the six-month follow-up.

The withdrawal of food or the interruption of meals has been effective in decreasing self-injurious behaviors in three profoundly retarded children (Lucero et al., 1976) and in the case of a blind, retarded eleven-year-old boy who persisted in hitting his head (Myers and Deibert, 1971).

Although these initially promising results reported for the use of punishment and aversive stimulation might tempt one to regard it as a panacea in an area which has enjoyed so little success at treatment, caution is required before assessing its efficacy.

Generalization of Effects

Although punishment may eliminate the self-injuring behavior in specific situations, this does not automatically extend to all other situations, including locale and persons. Severely retarded subjects have, for example, learned to discriminate between punishing adults and punishment versus nonpunishment locales (Bachman, 1972; Corte, Wolff, Locke, 1971). In this regard, Lovaas and Simmons (1969) have noted "the effect of shock appears specific to the situations in which it is administered" (p. 153). Moreover, the extent of generalization may depend on the patient's particular reinforcement history (Bucher and Lovaas, 1968).

Corte, Wolff, and Locke (1971) examined generalization in their treatment of a self-injuring retarded adolescent. Shock was administered, contingent on self-injuring in several situations (ward, cottage, treatment room) with the order of locales varying for each patient. They found little generalization to different situations or different experiments, although somewhat fewer shocks were required to eliminate the behavior in the second or third locales.

Merbaum (1973) also found it necessary to administer shock in several situations. His patient, an autistic, nonverbal twelve-year-old who beat his face with his fists, continued to self-injure in school and at home after such behavior had been eliminated in a treatment context. Introduction of shock (paired with no) delivered in the classroom, by teachers brought the rate of self-injury behavior to near zero with seventeen shocks. Since he continued to beat his face at home, his mother was trained in the use of contingent shock and reward of positive behavior resulting in the near elimination of the response at home as well. It is of note that the visible presence of the shock stick seemed to have a powerful deterrent effect in both these settings.

Singh (1976) also reports cases in which the problem of generalization was dealt with by having nursing staff and parents participate in the treatment program. A patient who chronically poked his eyes was punished by having his fingers tapped with a stick. As well, this was supplemented by a sixty-second time out upon self-injury and activity reinforces for five minutes when he did not injure himself. We cannot, of course, evalute which treatment component or combination produced supression in this case.

Generalization of supression was also a problem in the difficult case reported by Slawson and Davidson (1964). After the failure of traditional psychiatric treatments (supportive therapy, amytal interviews, tranquilizers, hypnosis, anaclitic therapy, insight therapy, and ECT) to deter a young woman from biting her tongue a behavior modification program was instituted. Verbal punishment by staff for tongue biting and praise for alternate behavior controlled the behavior in the presence of the staff. The young woman continued to bite her tongue while alone.

Bachman (1972) concluded that an adequate treatment program using aversive stimulation must involve the planned generalization of effects through administering the punishment in more than one situation and by more than one person.

Discriminability

The readily identifiable equipment typically used to administer shock (that is, a cattle prod) has been considered central to the problem of generalization of effects. Several authors have proposed shock delivery systems to counter these difficulties. Bachman (1972) suggests a remote control system, worn by the patient but controlled by a therapist in the general vicinity. The advantages he sees are in a less discriminable apparatus and therefore, presumably, greater generalization. Shock would not be specifically associated with the therapist. This would ensure generalization and counter the tendency to avoid the therapist. The immediacy of punishment would also be better controlled, and greater mobility would be allowed to the patient.

A variant of this system was designed and tested by Ball et al (1975). A nonrestraining jacket was equipped with a portable, battery-operated electrical pulse generator. Shock was activated by violent movement or impact on the part of the wearer. On tests with three retarded self-injuring patients, positive results were reported for two of them; the third apparently adapted to the shock. In addition to the advantages enumerated by Bachman, Ball and co-workers pointed out that the staff were thereby more available to focus on reward of positive behaviors. As well, they were able, in these cases, to fade out the use of the jacket for extended periods of time.

Wilbur, Chandler, and Carpenter (1974) developed a similar system for use with single, invariable self-injurious responses, like banging a specific body area. A contact switch was taped to the patient at the usual point of contact and connected to the shock delivery apparatus which was strapped to the patient. Contact activated the shock, which was delivered immediately. Using this apparatus they successfully treated several patients.

Merbaum (1973) found that the shock stick, which had been used to reduce the self-injurious behavior of a twelve-year-old male patient, acquired properties as a discriminative stimulus for punishment. The stick, although unused, was kept visible to the patient. Similar effects have been noted by Muttar et al. (1975), Tanner and Zeiler (1975), and Tate and Baroff (1966).

Side Effects

In his review of the use of aversive stimulation (response-contingent shock) Bachman (1972) concluded that no adverse side effects were apparent. In fact most authors reporting successful treatment through response-contingent shock report therapeutically positive side effects: the elimination of associated negative behaviors like crying, whining, and avoiding adults (Lovaas and Simmons, 1969; Tate and Baroff, 1966); and a spontaneous increase in positive behaviors like social responsiveness and alertness to the environment (Ball et al., 1975; Lovaas and Simmons, 1969; Merbaum, 1973; Muttar et al., 1975; Tate and Baroff, 1966; Wright, 1973).

In constrast, Jones, Simmons, and Frankel (1974) reported adverse effects for a child who had previously been treated by contingent shock with some success. A second contingent shock program nine months later was abandoned because the child's repertoire of self-injurious behavior expanded. Although the initial specific self-injurious response was decreasing, other forms had increased to the point of a net increase in self-injurious behavior. When this behavior was shocked as well, it increased; the original response reappeared and increased; the child refused to eat and had to be tube fed; and constant restraints were required.

Morrison (1972) also suggests that the use of shock must be approached with care due to the likelihood of suppressing responsiveness in general.

Habituation/Adaptation

Failure of treatment attributed to adaptation to shock is also reported. Ball et al. (1975), in tests of a shock jacket, report failure with one patient who adapted to shock. Stinnett and Hollender (1970) report the use of aversive stimulation as one of a variety of methods used in an attempt to control the severe eye banging of a young man. The patient carried a small shock device in the palm of his hand:

> . . . and it delivered a mild but unpleasant shock. The patient was instructed to press the button whenever he had the urge to hit his eye. He soon began to press the button ritualistically, but he continued to hit himself. [P. 372]

Tate (1972) described the case of an adolescent girl who had been in restraints for seven-and-a-half years for her self-mutilating behavior. He attributes the failure of aversive conditioning in this case to either the low intensity of the shock used or the interfering effects of drugs which the girl was receiving. Some therapists choose high intensity painful shock in order to ensure an effect, reasoning that the self-mutilator has developed a considerable tolerance for pain (for example, Lovaas and Simmons, 1969).

Persistence of the Effects

The persistence of the suppression of self-injurious behaviors following the application of this treatment modality has been reported as maintained from several months to a year or more. However, some reports would indicate a more gradual recovery in many patients (Ball et al., 1975; Tanner and Zeiler, 1975; Tate, 1972; Wright, 1973).

To a large extent, the durability of suppression is likely to be dependent on the contingencies in the daily living environment of the patient after the treatment program has been terminated. For this reason, the advisability of including positive reinforcement of other behavior in any program, particularly where shock is used, has been pointed out by many investigators (Bachman, 1972; Ball et al., 1975; Merbaum, 1973; Muttar et al. 1975; Singh, 1976; Tate, 1972; Tate and Baroff, 1966; Wilbur, Chandler, and Carpenter, 1974). This has been most poignantly stated by Lovaas and Simmons (1969):

> If the child had to go to such extremes as self-destruction to gain some attention from his attending adults, then it seems but reasonable that these adults, unless they were taught to respond to more appropriate behavior, would repeat themselves and start shaping some similarly alarming behavior. [P. 56]

The impact of the posttreatment environment is further illustrated by Tate's (1972) remarks, on discovering three years later a patient, successfully treated after seven-and-a-half years in restraints, once again spending most her day in restraints.

> Probably spontaneous recovery occurred one day and a new attendant on the ward, or possibly another patient, unfortunately reinforced it with attention and misguided "loving kindness". [P. 140]

As we have observed, the environment of the self-mutilator provides strong support for the maintenance of the behavior. As Ferster (1968) has noted, such behavior generates a kind of aversive effect on those around the mutilator, rendering it impossible not to react vigorously. Risley (1968) has noted the acquisition of intrinsically reinforcing properties with self-harming behavior, making them more difficult to deal with by external consequences only. Lovaas et al. (1965) have pointed out that the withdrawal of reinforcements can serve as a discriminative stimuli for the recurrence of self-destructive behavior since, in the past, self-destructive behavior has been associated with the reinstatement of reinforcement.

In sum, the persistence or durability of the treatment effects appear to depend upon the alternative contingencies in the posttreatment environment that serve to maintain suppression and reduce the opportunity for spontaneous recovery of the self-destructive behavior.

Finally the persistence of effects requires that the posttreatment environment provide the person with sufficient alternative avenues to meet the needs which initially prompted and subsequently maintained the self-injuring repertoire. This point is succinctly summarized by Peterson and Peterson (1968):

> Thus, self-destructive behaviors may be maintained because they control the behaviors of those in the child's milieu. The strength of self-destructive behaviors, then, may be partially dependent on the presence and effectiveness of alternate behaviors which can be used to influence the environment. [P. 304]

Ethical Issues

The research described in these reports indicates that the decision to use aversive control or punishment was arrived at only in the face of failure with more positive methods. The issue, however, has engendered considerable controversy among investigators (Ball, 1968; Bandura, 1969; Cohen, 1976; Lazarus, 1971). For those who react with horror at the suggestion of shocking children, Bachman (1972) offers the following palliative: "It [the electric shock] is probably . . . no more painful or traumatic than some injections, and is probably less brutal than electroconvulsive shock and psychosurgery" (p. 220). Parental permission was required and each therapist tried the shock himself before administering it. As well, Bachman contends, shock is never the only aspect of a treatment program. Desirable alternative behaviors are positively reinforced and punishment is eliminated once the self-injurious behavior is brought under control. Bachman concluded:

> . . . there is no good reason to permit children to severely injure themselves or to spend their early years in physical restraints;. . . a treatment program which combined the effective punishment of the deviant SIB with positive reinforcement of desirable, alternative responses would be the most efficient method of eliminating SIB. [P. 221]

We remain unconvinced by such arguments. However, Ball (1968) has pointed out the irony of well-meaning alternatives (such as tender loving care) having the demonstrated, albeit unwitting, potential for conditioning self-destructive behavior.

Both Bandura (1969) and Cohen (1976), in commenting on this controversy, have argued that the beneficial effects of this therapeutic regimen far outweigh the discomfort occasioned by aversion techniques. This position has been stated by Lazarus (1971):

> Just as a surgeon will assault and tear open one's flesh to save lives and alleviate suffering, an operant conditioner may use electric shock to prevent the head banging of autistic children who are bashing their heads to the point of damaging their brains, or biting their own fingers. [P. 205]

In conclusion, we agree with Bachman's (1972) review of the literature on aversive conditioning which concluded that none of the studies demonstrated that contingent shock per se eliminated the behavior.

The self-mutilating behaviors which have been treated by this technique are, almost without exception, those which occur with a high degree of frequency, such as self-slapping, head banging, scratching, and biting in autistic and retarded children. Its use with other populations and with other self-mutilatory behaviors such as carving is, to say the least, problematic if only because of its nonpublic and nonhabitual nature or the social-legal implications of the use of such nonvoluntary procedures in institutional settings.

Modeling and Assertiveness Training

Self-mutilation has often been viewed as an indirect expression of anger and hostility that the individual has been unable to express. In view of the popularity of the aggression-turned-inward hypothesis it is surprising that the literature contains only a few references to the use of assertiveness training as a technique for teaching the mutilator socially appropriate ways of expressing negative feelings such as irritation, resentment, and anger.

Cox and Klinge (1976) used a combination of assertiveness training and modeling in a multifaceted treatment for a self-burning patient. The therapist modeled appropriate responses to threatening situations which the patient typically avoided. He then reinforced the patient's appropriate social and anger responses and discouraged the patient from avoiding eye contact, talking softly, and using self-effacing remarks. The patient's self-mutilatory behavior stopped, and he continued to improve during the three-month follow-up.

Roback et al. (1972) included assertiveness training as one strategy in a complex approach to the successful treatment of a severe self-mutilating patient. They exercised appropriate caution in noting the difficulty in assessing the efficacy of any one component in this type of strategy.

Relaxation/Desensitization

In some instances self-mutilatory behavior may serve as an adaptive function by enabling the individual to avoid or escape from unpleasant situations or to avoid troubling or aversive thoughts that he cannot control. In such cases attempts at treatment might include procedures which train the patient to cope with the eliciting stimuli without having to resort to self-mutilation. Thus, Graff and Mallin (1967) successfully treated a self-cutter by holding her hand or cuddling her whenever she reported that she felt she was going to cut herself. Gardner and Gardner (1975) have also suggested that the mutilator should be trained in relaxation procedures in order that she might calm herself without resorting to self-mutilation when she experiences the increased level of tension which typically precipitates self-injury. Unfortunately, there is little evidence that relaxation training per se can be effective.

Ross, Meichenbaum, and Humphrey (1971) successfully treated an adolescent who had for many years banged her head against the bed at nights with such intensity that she woke herself up and disturbed the sleep of other patients on the ward. The patient also reported experiencing a recurrent nightmare in which she was assaulted by a man with a knife. It was hypothesized that the nightmare served as a stimulus for head banging, a response which served to wake her up and thereby terminate the distressing dream. The girl's head banging ceased following three weeks of desensitization during which she was trained to visualize successive parts of the dream while in a relaxed state. Relaxation training alone did not affect the head banging, but the desensitization procedure, following an initial increase, resulted in the elimination of head banging. The effect was maintained during a one-year follow-up.

Ernst (1973) reports on a patient who had a problem of nail-biting dating back to early childhood complicated by an intense compulsion to bite the inside of her mouth with extensive tissue damage. The patient used a gold wrist-counter to keep a daily count of the frequency of her biting. Following a baseline period, progressive relaxation training was initiated. The patient was taught to produce a relaxation response when cued by a signal from the wrist-counter. Relaxation training then focused on the jaw and lower facial areas. Ernst reported that the self-mutilative compulsion was controlled within four weeks. Improvement was maintained during a five-month follow-up.

Cautela and Baron (1973) described the successful application of a treatment regimen consisting of relaxation training to the severely self-injurious behavior of a twenty-year-old schizophrenic male patient. This patient's self-mutilatory behavior was always triggered by a compulsive thought that he must bite himself. The self-injury (eye poking, lip and tongue biting) ceased after three months and the improvement continued through discharge nine months later and at a two-year follow-up.

Similar counterconditioning procedures might be successfully applied to other self-mutilatory behaviors which serve to terminate or avoid aversive stimuli such as compulsive thoughts, fears, or hallucinations (Carr, 1977). This is an underdeveloped area of research. As we shall see in later chapters the notion that self-mutilation may represent a method whereby the patient gains a feeling of control over his environment has important implications for treatment. It suggests that therapy should aim to provide the patient with alternative means for controlling distressing thoughts or events or for coping with an environment which denies the individual a feeling that he can control his destiny.

Physical Restraint

Anyone faced with the intractibility of the determined self-mutilator will inevitably consider the use of physical restraint. We recall numerous occasions at Grandview, when, in the aftermath of a self-mutilatory episode, we found ourselves involved in serious discussion with colleagues, administrators, and staff regarding the development of preventive restraints. With some regularity the suggestions included straight jackets, splints, helmets, and a host of other devices, all designed to prevent further injury to the girl. Presented with similar frustrations, an amazing variety of devices have been developed and applied by clinicians to immobilize the mutilator and prevent further self-harm. The literature is replete with examples of nearly every conceivable method which one could imagine: to provide a buffer between the body of the mutilator and the tool or instrument of his mutilation or to prevent the mutilator from getting at the instrument or his own body through partial or total restraint. Such devices have included, helmets, face guards, gloves, straight jackets, wrist restraints, wood or cardboard splints tied around the mutilator's limbs, collars, or when all else fails, complete and total restraint by strapping them down to beds with an attendant providing around-the-clock surveillance (Azrin et al., 1975; Ball et al., 1975; Collins, 1964). Total restraint has been reported as lasting for over seven years in come cases (Tate, 1972).

As an example of one of the more exotic methods, Williams (1974) reported that the use of a fencing mask over a two-week period eliminated the self-destructive responses (to her face) of a young autistic woman. It was then possible to engage her in social activities.

It appears that a technology has developed in this field. Allen and Harris (1966) reported on the use of pneumatic splints as restraints in treatment of self-injurious behavior. Traditional restraint has involved immobilizing the patient by tying him down for extended periods of time. In contrast, "pneumatic restraints cover the limb, and when inflated, render the limb unbendable" (p. 320). Should the patient manage to hit himself, the blow is cushioned. The further advantages include the possibility of fading of restraints by reducing air pressure, enabling more mobility of limbs as treatment progresses. It is also said to provide some protection against injury during extinction procedures (Allen and Harris, 1966).

Contrary to the popular notion that the use of restraint indicates apathy and neglect, more often in this literature it serves as an index of the frustration and compassion of the clinician—frustration from the failure of their treatment repertoire and compassion in the desire to prevent further self-injury to their patient.

The use of restraint is of course fraught with difficulties, not the least of which is the underestimation of the ingenuity of the determined mutilator. Patients completely restrained and under constant surveillance have still managed to abrade their skin against the restraining device, use the restraint to constrict blood flow, hurl their bodies against objects, or even slip the restraints for the few seconds required to enucleate one of their eyes Tate (1972) has commented on the use of restraints in the management of children's self-injurious behavior. Tying the child to a bed or providing padding such as helmets or mittens may reduce injury, but it does not eliminate the behavior. It also has the distinct disadvantage of drastically reducing desirable behavior.

Restraint can also acquire reinforcing properties (Muttar et al., 1975; Saposnek and Watson, 1974; Tate, 1972), and the release from restraint can become a fear-eliciting and highly aversive event for a patient (Saposnek and Watson, 1974).

Finally, the use of restraint, isolation, and the requisite surveillance for such patients has a most undesirable set of potential consequences in institutional settings. Aside from the simple fact of its dubious efficacy in the elimination of self-injury, it can quickly become a treatment of choice, a control device reserved for the unruly or problematic patient resorted to with ever increasing frequency and selective application. Its use as a preventative device becomes ever more likely. Excess and abuse, we suggest, are an inevitable consequence of the use of restraint in institutional settings.

Conclusions

The literature on treatment of self-mutilation gives testimony to the fact that the ingenuity of therapists is only slightly exceeded by the ingenuity of the mutilator. Mutilators have been cuddled, loved, slapped, shocked, counseled, drugged, stimulated, isolated, reprimanded, and even lobotomized. In most instances we have very little convincing evidence that these interventions successfully prevent or ameliorate self-mutilation. Some, in fact, may augment the behavior. As Lovaas and Simmons (1969) have observed:

> The most common form of treatment consists of some combination of drugs and supportive, interpersonal therapy, and occasional electroconvulsive therapy. There is no evidence to demonstrate that any of these forms of treatment are effective. Conceivably some treatments could make the child worse. [P. 143]

The majority of the programs which appear to offer promise lack the methodological rigor that would enable us to attest to their efficacy. We do not wish to belabor the obvious shortcomings of field treatment and research.

Most treatment approaches can be described as eclectic or more accurately as a potpourri of trial and error. We should note, however, that because of the practical and ethical problems of conducting research on self-mutilation it is extremely difficult to separate out the factors which contribute to the success or failure of any approach.

The treatment programs we have described no doubt constitute a biased sample of treatment efforts. There are probably countless others which have not been published because they have failed.

The literature on self-mutilation is voluminous. The literature on its treatment is sparse. This may well be because self-mutilation is generally intractable to treatment. Cursory examination of the treatment literature can create a false impression that only the behavior modifiers are active in this area. Close examination reveals that there is actually a host of therapists from other schools who have attempted to treat the self-mutilators.

Treatment by the behavior modifier, because of his limited interest in causes of self-mutilation, is readily identified because of his focus on eliminating symptoms. Treatment conducted by other therapists is often embedded in descriptions of the psychodynamics of their patient's mutilation.

If the reader attends only to the behavioral approaches to treatment, he can be misled into thinking that the treatment of the self-mutilator can be rapidly effected by the application of some simple, straightforward conditioning technique. Some of the behavioral programs have enjoyed dramatic success with some patients. It is important to note that they have been almost exclusively limited to the treatment of a select sample of patients consisting of autistic and retarded children whose self-injurious acts represent only a small sample of the range of self-mutilatory behavior. It remains to be seen whether such techniques can (or should) be generalized to other populations and to the broader variety of self-injurious behavior.

Much more representative of treatment approaches in the literature is that found in a report by Slawson and Davidson (1964), who document the treatments which were sequentially applied to a tongue-biting patient: custodial care, psychotherapy, phenothiazines, faith healing, supportive staff therapy, amytal interviews, chlorpromazine, hypnosis, anaclitic therapy, educative therapy, electroconvulsive therapy, behavioral conditioning, out-patient psychotherapy, and trifuloperazine.

The patient continued to bite her tongue.

6 The "Carving Study"

The Riddle

In this chapter we return to the riddle we presented in chapter 1. There we stated that we had been successful three times in eliminating self-mutilation among the Grandview adolescents. For the sake of suspense we shall not tell you about the first time until later. That is only fair since at the time of our success we ourselves did not realize we had been successful.

To reiterate our riddle, the first time we eliminated self-mutilation we did not know we had done so, let alone how. The second time we knew we had been successful, but we did not know why. Much later we discovered, with a little help from our friends, why we had been successful the first two times. This was when we finally recognized that we had developed and had been unwittingly employing some unorthodox strategies in our work with the girls. Later, when we deliberately and systematically applied these strategies, we eliminated carving a third time.

Overview

As we reported earlier, when we arrived at Grandview we quickly learned the extent of the self-mutilation problem; of the 136 girls in the institution at that time 86 percent had carved their bodies at least once, and many had carved repeatedly. Only a few girls had never self-mutilated in this manner.

In order to try to understand this behavior, we did all the traditional things that the social scientist-professional is trained to do. We sought advice from the available literature. The three previous chapters document what we learned. We also observed and charted the phenomenon. Then we went directly to the girls to elicit information as to their perception of their carving. Our more informal talks with the girls led to the development of a structured interview. Through this interview we set out to obtain information on carving from the girls in a systematic fashion.

In the girls' account of their carving behavior they frequently made reference to social factors which were seen as important in the motivation of their self-mutilation. Accordingly, we made a careful study of some social-situational variables through sociometric analysis of the girls' peer relations. Next, partly because of our clinical training, we investigated possible personality correlates of self-mutilation by administering a standard instrument which is commonly used with populations of this type: the Minnesota Multiphasic Personality Inventory (MMPI). The MMPI, it was thought, would give us some insight as to the degree and nature of the psychopathology we presumed to be associated with carving.

Based on some of our initial findings, one explanation that occurred to us was that self-mutilation represented an interaction between psychopathology and social adaptation. Therefore, we decided to examine the relationship between carving and other indicants of acting-out behavior as measured by frequency of escape attempts and recidivism. In this chapter we present the results of our research referred to as the carving study.

Sample

The participants ranged in age from twelve to seventeen, the majority being between fourteen and sixteen years. The distribution of IQs at the school was essentially normal, but there was a marked academic retardation in the population (median retardation: 1.8 yrs; mean grade level: seventh grade). All girls had been screened in a reception unit, and none carried a diagnosis indicating the presence of either brain damage or thought disorder. The girls were admitted to the training school for an indeterminate period following their adjudication in juvenile court. They demonstrated a variety of behavior problems such as habitual truancy, alcohol and drug abuse, running away from home, and unacceptable or aberrant sexual behavior. Most were admitted as unmanageable, and the majority had previous appearances in juvenile court, many having been unsuccessfully placed on probation or in foster homes or other residential settings.

Carving, as we have noted, was a term employed by the girls. It represents a form of self-mutilation which we have classified as cutting. In order to avoid confusion we will use the term carving to refer only to the behavior of the girls at Grandview.

From the school's total population, ninety-six girls agreed to participate in our initial study of carving. From this group seventy-one girls completed all of the required information. The data from the other fifteen girls were discarded because of subsequent refusals to participate or insufficient data. The final group studied consisted of fifteen girls who had never carved, fifteen girls who had carved only once, and forty-one girls who had carved more than once. The girls who had carved reported 500 separate carvings. The average number of carvings was 8.9 per girl with a range of 1 to 33.

Body Charts

Each girl was asked to complete a body chart indicating the location and nature of each of her carvings. Although it had been customary at the institution during weekly medical checks to conduct body inspections for evidence of carving, it was decided to avoid this kind of investigation for research purposes because we viewed it as humiliating for the girls. Additionally, we wished to avoid giving undue attention to the carvings. Because some of this behavior might be motivated by attention seeking, to do so might exacerbate the problem.

The data obtained are self-report data, but since the vast majority of carvings were clearly visible on the girls' legs or arms, simple observation served as a check on the reliability of their reports.

The body charts were classified by independent raters in terms of composition and referents. Some of the carvings were simple scratches (3.2 percent). Others (12.2 percent) entailed complex statements such as, in hell at sixteen, or to mom, with all my hate, 71 percent were names or initials, 36 percent of these referring to the girl's lovelight. *Lovelight* was a term used to refer to a girl friend in the institution. Lovelight relationships were frequently intimate and intense, though not necessarily sexual, and were often short-lived. These relationships were part of a pseudokinship system which developed in the institution over many years. It was a complex system which incorporated family units in which girls were identifed as other girl's training school mom, dad, sister, or brother, and behaved according to their labels. Similar pseudofamilies have been reported in other correctional institutions for females (Foster, 1975; Taylor, 1965). Love-lighting, in our view, provided the girl with the advantage of being emotionally attached to a peer without the necessity of an overt homosexual relationship.

Table 6-1
Classification and Referent of Carving
(data expressed as percentage of total number of carvings: 500)

	Names	*Initials*	*Words or Phrases*	*Mixed*	*Scratches*	*Designs*	*Other*	*Total*
Lovelight	14.4	18.2		3.8				36.4
Mother	7.8	0.8		2.2				10.8
Other family	10.8	1.8		1.0				13.6
Boyfriends	5.6	6.6		1.2				13.4
Girlfriends outside the institution	0.6	1.4						2.0
Other	2.0	1.6	12.2	2.6	3.2	2.0	0.2	23.8
Total	41.2	30.4	12.2	10.8	3.2	2.0	0.2	100

Table 6-2
Frequency of Carving by Area of Body

	Legs	*Arms*	*Face*	*Stomach*	*Breasts*
Frequency	252	204	22	13	9
Percentage	50.4	40.8	4.4	2.6	1.8

Table 6-1 presents the carving data according to composition and referent. Of the 500 carvings 78 percent had no apparent emotional content other than what might be inferred from the fact that a girl had carved her lovelight's or her mother's name or initial. Rating of the emotional content of the remaining 107 carvings revealed that 56 percent expressed love; 28 percent, hate or anger; 10 percent, sadness; 5 percent, guilt; and 1 percent, love-hate ambivalence.

The girls most frequently carved their legs and arms: 50 percent and 40 percent of the carvings, respectively. The face, stomach, and breasts followed in frequency in that order and accounted for the balance of the carvings, as indicated in Table 6-2. Facial carving, which was particularly disfiguring, occurred infrequently and was done only by multiple carvers. In no instance did it occur in the case of a girl who had not been described in reports on file as "very attractive."

Structured Interview

A structured interview to provide information about carving and the girl's feelings about it was conducted with each participant. Although one-third of the girls reported having heard of carving before admission to training school, no girl had carved prior to being institutionalized. Since the majority of the girls had long-term experience in delinquent subcultures, we felt that this form of self-mutilation (carving) must be somewhat institution-bound rather than being a phenomenon commonly found within delinquent groups in community settings. However, we have recently received reports of the same phenomenon occurring in community group homes.

The participants classified their initial feelings toward carving as good, neutral, or stupid. Over 80 percent reported that when first hearing of carving (usually in the reception unit of the training school) they thought it was a stupid thing to do. Of the girls who later carved, 75 percent had changed their minds and no longer thought it was foolish. Interestingly, in spite of their changed opinion, the majority of these girls expressed an interest in having their carving removed surgically.

The majority of the carvers (75 percent) reported that they had done so when either angry or depressed. In the majority of instances (70 percent) the girls were alone when they carved, either in segregation or in their room. Group carving was not common and only rarely did one girl carve with another girl. In the girls' opinion, when asked why other girls carve, most (48 percent) reported that carving was done to please lovelight. Specifically, they reported that carving served several different purposes related to the lovelight system:

1. a demonstration of affection
2. a sealing of a pact
3. a demonstration of anger or hurt engendered by their lovelight rejecting them
4. a means of retaliating when the lovelight's behavior engendered their jealousy
5. a manipulation designed to force their lovelight to pay some attention to them

Examination of the girls' reports of methods of carving makes it clear that security measures to control their access to sharp instruments such as razor blades or knives are likely to be a singularly ineffective preventive strategy. Although such instruments were used, the girls more frequently used broken bobby pins or needles and pins smuggled out of sewing class. Moreover, we learned that many other objects could be used, including plaster chipped off walls, pens or pencils, broken glass or china, wood splinters from furniture, strands of hair used as a saw, the metal ends of shoe laces, nails gouged out of shoes or furniture, or broken-off fingernails.

The majority of girls (51 percent) reported that carving involved no pain, whereas 31 percent reported slight pain and 18 percent extreme pain. When they experienced pain, most girls reported they simply stopped cutting for a while, then carried on. Of the carvers 29 percent reported feeling satisfied immediately after carving, 22 percent felt stupid, and 11 percent sad. A variety of feelings were reported by the remaining 38 percent. In the vast majority of instances the carving was viewed by one or more people soon after the incident even when the girl claimed she wanted to keep it hidden. Seventy-five percent of the girls reported having done nothing at all to hide the carving or to attempt to avoid being caught and punished.

When asked to suggest how carving could be prevented, the multicarvers suggested increased recreational activities (34 percent), eliminating the lovelight system (19 percent), and having someone to talk to (10 percent). Some (20 percent) had no suggestions, and others (17 percent) argued that there was nothing the staff could do to prevent carving.

Sociometric Measure

Each subject completed a questionnaire which consisted of fourteen items. Ten items were designed to indicate each subject's preference for other girls who were in the study. Each girl selected from the total list of participants her first, second, and third choice of a girl she would choose in a variety of categories, for example, a companion, close friend, or roommate. Four items were designed to tap the power structure in the residences at the training school. These questions required a participant to indicate which girl they thought was the "sharpest" in their residence, and which girl they thought the other girls and the staff viewed as the "sharpest." A sociometric score for each girl was obtained by assigning 3 points for each first choice she received, 2 for each second choice, and 1 for each third choice. Scores for each girl were corrected to equate for the number of girls in the various residences. The corrected sociometric scores ranged from 0 to 260 with a mean of 52.84 and a median of 36.

The data clearly suggest that the girls who do not carve themselves are chosen less frequently and are not, in the eyes of their peers, the "sharpest" girls in the institution. The average sociometric scores for the fifteen noncarvers and the fifty-six carvers are 25 and 64, respectively. This difference is statistically significant ($F = 3.92$; 1.69 $df; p < .05$).

MMPI

The results of an MMPI which had been administered to each girl were compared for the three carving groups: fifteen noncarvers, fifteen single carvers, and forty-one multicarvers. The means for all groups on ten of the sixteen scales tended to fall near the means of the standardization population (within 1.5 standard deviations). On six of the scales, however, the means were abnormally elevated: D, depression; Pd, psychopathic deviate; Pa, paranoia; F, validity score; Sc, schizophrenia; and Ma, hypomania.

In each instance, the means for the single-carving group were substantially closer to the standardization mean than were the means for either of the other two groups. On two of the scales (F and Sc) the difference in means was statistically significant ($p < .05$). This analysis, then, appeared to suggest that the girls who carved once were more "normal" than the multicarvers. But they also appeared to be more "normal" than girls who did not carve at all.

In order to test the possibility that the single-carving groups was more "normal" than the other two groups, the latter were pooled into a single group and another analysis was done. No mean difference between multicarvers and noncarvers was statistically significant. The results of this anaylsis are presented in table 6-3. It can be seen that the single carvers scored lower on each scale than did the noncarvers and multicarvers, and significantly lower on three scales: F, D, and Sc.

Table 6–3
Analysis of MMPI Data on Six Scales for Single Carvers vs. Noncarvers and Multicarvers

MMPI Scale	*Single Carvers* $\bar{X}$	*Noncarvers and Multicarvers* $\bar{X}$	*F*	$p<$
F	68.5	75.1	7.0	.009
D	55.2	61.5	3.9	.04
Pd	76.4	81.4	2.6	.10
Pa	69.6	76.1	2.5	.11
Sc	73.0	84.0	6.1	.01
Ma	69.1	74.2	3.2	.07

The fact that the single carvers scored lower on the F scale, a validity scale of the MMPI, suggests that the differences obtained on the other five scales were merely a function of the other two groups' less valid performance. However, Carson (1960), has suggested an alternative hypothesis. The means of both groups fall between 65 and 80. This is the range which Carson found to be "indicative of unusual or markedly unconventional thinking . . . frequently [appearing] in sullen, rebellious personalities of the schizoid, antisocial or 'Bohemian' type" (p. 5). Thus, either the single carvers were more honest and cooperative in completing the MMPI or were less sullen, rebellious, schizoid, and antisocial. Either factor may be indicative of a delinquent characteristic. Following this reasoning it can be tentatively suggested that single carvers are significantly less delinquent than noncarvers and multicarvers.

Elevation on the F, D, Pd, and Sc scales represents a "basic schizoid configuration" (Carson, 1960). Elevated scores on the Pa scale, when associated with this schizoid configuration, are indicative of "angry, sullen people who utilize excessively a transfer of blame mechanism. Typically they are rigidly argumentative and difficult in social relations" (p. 130). When the Ma-scale scores are also elevated, as is the case with the noncarvers and multicarvers, it is reasonable to expect personalities characterized by acting-out, antisocial, and criminal behavior, an inordinate need for excitement, and a tendency toward aggression. The mean Ma-scale score of the noncarvers and multicarvers is in the range where "there is increasing likelihood of maladaptive hyperactivity, irritability, and insufficient inhibitory capacity" (p. 21).

The MMPI data indicate that the girls who had carved only once were, as a group, significantly more socially facile than were the noncarvers and multicarvers. As a group the single carvers are more able to relate positively to other people, less prone to act in a hostile and aggressive fashion, and more able to control their impulses and to accept the responsibility for the consequences of their behavior. In short, the mean scores of the noncarver and multicarver groups were much more suggestive of pathology. The girls who had carved only once appeared to be less seriously disturbed or delinquent than those who either had not carved at all or had carved more than once.

Individual Pathology or Social Adaptation?

These results led us to wonder whether the carving of our girls can be considered to be an expression of psychopathology, or alternatively, whether it may be a sort of initiation rite, the performance of which indicates that the girl has identified with the subculture and as such is a candidate for peer group approval and social reinforcement.

As we saw in chapter 4, previous investigators of self-mutilation have tended to emphasize one or another of two contrasting positions; their explanations have been essentially uni-dimensional, their choice seemingly reflective of the characteristics of their sample (institution versus clinic) or their theoretical orientation (psychodynamic versus social learning). However, by itself each of these explanations has difficulty accounting for the data presented above. If carving is an expression of psychopathology, it is difficult to explain why the single carvers scored lower on the MMPI scales than the noncarvers. If carving is essentially a social phenomenon, a behavior that yields social approval from peers, it is difficult to explain why multicarvers are socially preferred less frequently than single carvers. Social reinforcement does not appear to be a linear function of self-mutilation.

An alternative explanation of these data is that carving represents an interaction between psychopathology and social adaptation. The adolescents who had carved themselves but had done so only once appeared to be the least disturbed girls in the institution but also the most socially accepted. One explanation proposed is that these girls had carved in order to identify with the subculture. Once having done so, their minimal degree of disturbance made it possible for them to perceive the situational reality and stop mutilating themselves. One instance of carving behavior appears to have been sufficient to identify them in the eyes of their peers as belonging. This minimum of self-mutilatory conforming behavior appears to be sufficient for this group.

In contrast, the noncarvers received fewer sociometric choices than did the other groups. This evidence contradicts the verbal reports of the noncarvers who felt that failing to carve was not causing them to be socially isolated. This is exactly the type of alienation and misperception of reality that the MMPI findings would lead us to expect to find in this group of girls. Their failure to carve does not appear to have stemmed from any sort of essential health, but rather from a personality disturbance that manifested itself in depression, withdrawal, and autistic-like thinking. They are nonparticipants in social activity, carving included.

The group of multicarvers was less homogenous than the other groups. More disturbed and less frequently chosen than the single carvers, they may be represented as those who were expressing their pathology in a way apparently sanctioned by the subculture with which they identified. This group included those girls who presumably failed to recognize that they could stop carving themselves and still maintain their social position and also those who failed to comprehend that this type of behavior was, of itself, not enough to gain social approval.

The essence of the above discussion is that it is not a presence or absence of carving that indicates degree of personality dysfunction. It is rather the amount of this type of behavior that an individual displays and the purpose that it is serving for her. Carving has a U-shaped relationship with emotional disturbance in institutionalized delinquents. Those girls who display none of the behavior and those who display a great deal of it appear to be significantly more disturbed than those who utilize these types of behavior in moderation.

Femininity

There is one finding which we wish to highlight. On one MMPI scale the groups were almost identical: the masculinity-femininity (Mf) scale. Self-mutilators were not different in femininity than non-self-mutilators. This finding raises some questions about interpretations of self-mutilatory behavior in terms of a notion of a predominantly feminine form of self-punitive behavior or masochism.

Escape

Our data suggested to us that self-mutilatory behavior was neither simply an expression of pathology nor simply a social phenomenon. Rather, we reasoned, self-mutilatory behavior may be a function of the interaction between a girl's personality and the social reinforcements that she seeks and receives within a training school setting. Accordingly, it was hypothesized that other forms of deviant behavior that are frequently shown by institutionalized delinquents should tend to correlate positively with self-mutilatory behavior. It has already been shown that the largest percentage of carvings are related to the lovelight system. This suggests, though not in any conclusive manner, that the girls who exhibited a great deal of self-mutilatory behavior were also more involved with the institution's pseudohomosexual system. In order to see if there is a relationship between types of antisocial behavior, it was decided to count the number of escape attempts (successful or unsuccessful) that a girl made while a ward of the training school. Specifically, it was hypothesized that the number of escapes that a girl attempted would positively correlate with the number of carvings that she reported. It was further hypothesized that the group of noncarvers, because of the withdrawn, dissociated nature of their disturbance, would have tended to try to escape least often. The prediction was also made that the single carvers would show a low incidence of escape attempts because of their more realistic appraisal of their situation. Similarly, the multicarvers would tend to escape more frequently because they were less appreciative of the reality consequences of their behavior and also more inclined toward acting-out.

It appears that a relationship did exist between types of acting-out behavior. A positive correlation ($r = .44$) was found between a number of carvings and number of escape attempts. This correlation was significant ($Z = 3.68; p < .0001$, one-tailed test).

In order to test the second part of this hypothesis, that the noncarvers and single carvers would have attempted fewer escapes than the multicarvers, the data was arranged on the 2x3x2 matrix shown in table 6-4.

The seventy-one girls who participated in the study were responsible for 107 escape attempts or a mean of 1.51 attempts per girl. It was found that forty-three of these seventy-one girls, or 61 percent, had engaged in less than the mean number of attempts. The expected number of girls in each below-mean cell is $.61x$. The column total and the expected number of girls in each "Above-Mean" cell is $.39x$. Inspection of table 6-4 shows that the observed frequencies differ from the expected frequencies in the directions predicted. These differences are statistically significant (chi square = $6.24; p < .05$). Thus we are able to conclude that there was a significant relationship between number of carves and number of escape attempts; multicarvers attempted to escape more frequently than single carvers and noncarvers.

Table 6-4
Expected and Obtained Frequencies of Escape Attempts in Noncarvers, Single carvers, and Multicarvers

	Noncarvers		*Single carvers*		*Multicarvers*		
Below Mean	E=9	0=12	E=9	0=11	E=25	0=20	43
Above Mean	E=6	0=3	E=6	0=4	E=16	0=21	26
Total	15		15		41		71

Recidivism

Following their release from the training school each girl was followed up for two years to determine whether she was returned to the institution because of unsatisfactory community adjustment. Information was obtained on all but one girl, a multicarver who was committed to a psychiatric hospital.

The amount of carving that a girl had done in the institution before her release did not appear to be related to whether or not she became a recidivist. Excluding the multicarver who was committed to the psychiatric hospital, the mean number of carvings for all girls while in the institution was 7.04. Exactly 40 percent of each group were returned to the training school at least once because of unsatisfactory adjustment in the community during the two-year follow-up. Neither the recidivists with a mean of 7.10 carves nor the nonrecidivists with an average of 7.00 carves differed significantly from the grand mean. This form of self-mutilation is unrelated to recidivism.

To sum up, two conclusions seem to be appropriate to these data. First, self-mutilation of this type is not a simple or direct manifestation of psychopatholgy. There is, in fact, a U-shaped relationship. Multicarvers do not differ in terms of personality disturbance from noncarvers, and single carvers are emotionally healthier than both of these groups.

Second, carving cannot be explained by a simple social adaptation model. Social approval is not a linear function of the frequency of carving. Girls who carved on a single occasion were more popular than girls who carved frequently or not at all. Social factors are undoubtedly operative, but carving is not simply a method of gaining social acceptance.

Traditional Remedies

As part of the carving study we examined the history of the institution in terms of its response to the self-mutilatory behavior of its residents. We suspect that the remedies for self-mutilation that Grandview has tried are not much different from those attempted by other institutions.

As we noted, a considerable variety of intervention strategies had been used over the years with girls who had carved themselves. Among these were punishing carving with loss of privileges, restricting the carver's choice of clothing to articles which hid the scars, extra work, removal of the carver from group activities, solitary confinement, close and individualized supervision, increased length of stay in the institution, absence of visitors, chemotherapy, lecturing, threatening, counseling. Increased recreational activity, particularly of a physical nature, had also been tried.

Regrettably, no concurrent systematic analysis had been provided as to the effects of such treatment efforts, and we must rely on anecdotal reports. We assume that the longevity of each of the above remedies is testimony to their efficacy.

The present study, at first glance, appears to affirm the effectiveness of the institution's traditional remedies: approximately 21 percent of this sample of girls never carved and 21 percent ceased carving after one episode. Perhaps we can assume that the institution's remedies discouraged many potential carvers from carving and dissuaded one-time carvers from persisting in this behavior. We rather doubt that such is the case. We are more persuaded that these girls seldom carved for reasons other than those related to the institution's remedies. Our interpretation of the present data is that there are many girls who, after one episode of self-mutilation had gained them social acceptance, would cease carving regardless of whether their self-mutilatory behavior was punished.

Even assuming the efficacy of the foregoing interventions, it is clear that they are ineffective with a large number of girls–21 percent of the sample carved at least once and an additional 58 percent carved more than once (an average of 11.8 times for multicarvers). Further evidence of limited effectiveness is the fact that carving persisted as a problem for many years. The remedies may have served to dissuade some girls from persisting in such behavior, but they were not effective as a deterrent for a large number of residents at this institution. Generalizing from our sample, they were an ineffective deterrent for some 79 percent of the population.

Most of the remedies took the form of aversive consequences–punishment. We would hypothesize that punishment may not only be an ineffective deterrent to such behavior but may actually engender carving in at least two ways:

1. Punishment signals to these adolescents that carving is disapproved by the adults in the institution, and therefore, the peer group can use its occurrence as an initiation rite into an antisocial culture. Our view is that these adolescents would evaluate it more negatively and encourage it less if it did not elicit such strong negative reactions in adults.
2. Punishment of carving provides attention and recognition. A single carver may decide that the attention and status gained by carving did not justify the disfigurement it produced. However, spectators, including girls who have not carved and multicarvers, may see the attention as well worth working for. This ripple effect is an important consideration in behavior which is as contagious as carving. Because of the abhorrent quality of skin cutting, it tends to evoke a strong response of concern–on the part of both staff and girls–which an onlooker may misinterpret as sympathy but which the carver more properly perceives as condemnatory. Each incident could become a cause celebre which would then have the potential for triggering an outburst of carving. Punishment, then, may prevent recurrence in a perpetrator (we doubt it does) but may stimulate it in many others.

Some punishing events, such as social isolation and room confinement, may actually encourage carving by creating the opportunity for its occurrence.

Reflections

We should note at this point that we were gratified, perhaps even surprised, by the reaction of the girls to our research. Unlike the sometimes recalcitrant college students or albino rats which had more frequently been the object of our research pursuits, these subjects were enthusiastic, interested, and eager participants. We had no difficulty in eliciting information from the girls about their carving behavior. They gave us answers to questions we had not asked or even thought of asking. As we showed interest in their views we were deluged with details about their institutional life and the circumstances surrounding carving and its significance to them.

Given the significance of our findings and the enthusiastic contributions of our participants, we were more than a little angered and disappointed by the negative attitude of the institution's administrative director. We were "called on the carpet" and told abruptly, decisively, and in no uncertain terms that we had no business conducting such research. The administrator was appalled that we had undertaken the research without seeking his permission. More distressing to him was that, as he viewed it, we had arranged to have researchers running around the institution asking questions and getting the girls excited about carving. His distress was, of course, appropriate for two reasons. First, it was assumed (incorrectly as we later found out) that giving the girls attention for their carving would quickly lead to an epidemic of carving. Second, he did not want to broadcast the fact that such behaviors were occurring in his institution. His anxiety about the possible adverse effects to the institution of such publicity represented a realistic fear. After all, it was a public institution run by a government department. In the legislature, if it were known that government wards were mutilating themselves, the opposition might mutilate the government. The administrator was in an extremely difficult position. He was faced with severely behavior-disordered adolescents who were continually defacing their bodies by self-mutilation, and try as he might, he was absolutely unable to do anything about it. Here we were, as he put it, a group of ivory-towered academics who had no better ideas on how to stop the self-mutilation than he did, and we were going to "tell the world." "But," we protested, "it is the researcher's ethical obligation to communicate his results." Quite. If the ethical problems of research were that simple we would have no need for ethics.

Later, when we discussed our intention to resign and verbalized our frustration and anger, it gradually occurred to us, with the able help of an insightful assistant administrator, that our concern was about professional power and academic freedom, not the welfare of the girls. Our best course of action if we were as interested in helping as we were about publishing would be to use our resources and our brains to help the institution find some way of treating the girls so that they might not resort to carving themselves. We were co-opted into joining the administrators in their efforts to deal with self-mutilation rather than opposing their control of our professional freedom.

We were refused permission to publish and promptly forgot about the study.

7 In Search of a Panacea

Trials and Tribulations

In this chapter we describe the results of our examination of the effectiveness of a number of treatment modalities in reducing the frequency of carving at Grandview. Our treatment research was conducted over a long period of time in sequential phases. In each phase a new experimental treatment program was introduced based on hypotheses developed from the observations and results obtained in previous phases. This approach enabled us to improve our intervention strategies with new groups of girls based on our evaluation of the accumulated wisdom of preceding treatment programs.

When we learned of the adminstration's response to the carving study we retreated to the sanctum of our offices to lick our wounds and to enjoy the comfortable sinecure of psychological testing and report writing.

Several months later we were drawn back into the fray. We returned somewhat reluctantly and with diminishing memory of past frustrations. This was the beginning of a search for a means of treating these apparently intractable girls that would lead us through disappointment, frustration, and anguish that may never be neutralized by our final success. Our reentry occurred when the government decided to convert one of the residence units at Grandview into a psychiatric center. An impressive cadre of highly qualified professionals, including psychiatrists, social workers, psychologists, and special education teachers, were employed, and they introduced an intensive treatment program. Each girl received individual psychotherapy, and each was involved in group psychotherapy with highly competent therapists. The total milieu was mobilized into a therapeutic environment. Staff training for all personnel was extensive. It was an impressive program geared to the traditional psychiatric approach. Ten girls selected from the total population because of the severity and persistence of their behavior problems were transferred to the new unit and were involved in the program.

Most of the explanations of carving which were in vogue at that time were based on psychodynamic notions. Psychotherapy in a treatment milieu appeared to be the most appropriate intervention approach. Unfortunately its effectiveness did not match its promise. Our treatment program only augmented the girls' behavior problems. The detailed results of our treatment programs are reported elsewhere (Ross, 1977; Ross and McKay, 1976a,b, 1978). Suffice it to say, psychodynamically oriented therapy in an intensive treatment milieu increased carving more than tenfold.

It is clear that one must be cautious in interpreting this outcome. The intensive milieu treatment program was conducted without experimental controls. It suggests, however, that treatment of self-mutilation has potential for harm as well as for good.

Pilot Behavior Modification Program

If we view carving as a learned response, an instrumental act that has some rewarding effect, then the treatment of choice would be behavior modification, specifically operant conditioning.

While we were becoming increasingly distressed by the increase in the girls' carving in the intensive treatment milieu program, we became aware of the work that was being done by behavior modifiers with retardates and schizophrenics in various institutions. These programs appeared to be enjoying remarkable success with a wide range of behavioral problems. At that time behavior modification was a relatively untried approach with offenders. Schwitzgebel (1969) had conducted his streetcorner behavior modification research with delinquents in the Boston slums, and Cohen and Philipczack (1971) were utilizing programmed learning and behavioral techniques in a correctional institution in Washington, D.C. There had also been some laboratory experiments with offender subjects (Burchard and Tyler, 1965; Tyler, 1967).

Enamored with the promise of behavior modification we developed a token economy for the ten girls whose behavior had been deteriorating so badly under the previous treatment regimen. The token economy was an elementary one, the first of its kind to be tried with female offenders.

The staff rated each girl's behavior on a 12-point scale. Good behavior earned the girls poker chips. The better the girls behaved, the more poker chips they earned. With the chips they could purchase goods such as cosmetics and clothes, and privileges, such as trips and dances. Without poker chips they led a spartan existence. The staff were thoroughly trained in the principles and techniques of reinforcement therapy. In effect they were asked to reward good behavior and to avoid reinforcing misbehavior (including carving).

We obtained dramatic and long-lasting improvement in the girls' behavior. Within five weeks of the introduction of treatment most of their behavior problems had almost disappeared. Self-mutilation, including carving, was eliminated. Control of the girls' behavior was maintained through the five-month period prior to their release from the institution. Finally, a promise had been realized.

This is one of the three times we eliminated self-mutilation.

Obviously this treatment program provided only crude evidence for the effectiveness of behavior modification strategy. However, the effect was so impressive that, coupled with the acclaim which the behavior modification movement was enjoying generally, it generated enthusiasm for this approach and justified the expansion of this type of behavioral programming into a long-term treatment-research project.

Phase 1 Behavior Modification Program

The institution's directors also became caught up in the wave of popularity of behavior modification and, encouraged by the remarkable success of our efforts, urged us to expand our program. We began to provide service for two units of a fifty-bed facility in the institutional complex. In allowing ourselves to be persuaded, we subtly wrested the actual, though unofficial, control of the unit from the administrators. We did so because we realized that in order to conduct behavioral intervention adequately one has to control the environment. We managed to gain this control by gradually persuading the administrators to convert to a behavior modification approach most of the institution's rules and regulations, as well as its systems of dispensing or withholding commodities and privileges. The management of the institution came under our control as we subtly engineered the nature of all the contingencies between the offenders' behavior and the staff's response to these behaviors. The total environment was modified such that its programs and practices came to be determined by reinforcement principles. Although we stopped short of structural change, we transformed the institution dramatically. Some of the problems involved in engendering such change are described elsewhere (Ross and McKay, 1978a; Ross and Price, 1976).

The remarkable outcome of the pilot behavior modification program had persuaded the Ontario Mental Health Foundation to lend generous financial support to extend our research into a long-term investigation of the efficacy of applying behavior modification techniques with adolescent offenders.

In our research design, the sequential nature of our project prevented us from using random assignment of subjects to the various treatment and control groups. However, we were able to select from the population of offenders we treated (over two hundred girls) comparison groups of subjects matched on a variety of factors deemed important: age, length of institutionalization, and IQ. There were no pretreatment differences in the institutional behavior of participants in different treatment or control groups.

The program was monitored on a continuing basis by obtaining data on each girl's institutional and postinstitutional adjustment. These data led us to introduce major changes in our program from time to time in an attempt to improve treatment outcome.

We were able to add several behavioral engineers and research assistants to our staff of therapists. At the introduction of our expanded token economy we had, in addition to psychiatric and social work staff, more than twenty members on our treatment-research team. Our team provided staff training, sometimes on an around-the-clock basis, for some thirty-five teachers and supervisors (matrons) of the girls. We located some of our research staff directly in the maximum security unit which housed many of the most behaviorally disordered adolescent girls in the Province of Ontario. Some of our staff used cells as offices. From that base our influence extended into virtually every part of the institution and into every aspect of the girls' lives. We ran the institution. Perhaps the institution ran us.

Incidentally, while our large-scale behavior modification program was being planned, we exerted a great deal of energy trying to persuade the officials to improve the environment in the institution in order to provide a more homelike and humane atmosphere in hopes of reducing self-mutilation. We were successful in many ways in breaking through much of the paramilitary atmosphere. For example, we enabled some of the girls to wear their own clothes instead of the institutional uniform; we developed an improved recreation program; we lobbied for more youthful and male staff; we promoted student government through councils and committees; and we increased parental contacts. Even the drab monochromatic institutional decor was modified as the girls received permission to decorate their surroundings. We provided them modern teaching and entertainment devices such as stereos, teaching machines, and videotapes. They also had an abundance of cosmetics, clothing, and lingerie. We arranged for visiting rock groups, dancing partners, arts and crafts programs, games, and trips. They were remembered on their birthdays with personal gifts—a somewhat unique occurrence in institutional settings.

All of these environmental improvements had no apparent effect whatsoever on the frequency of self-mutilation. The girls used their new recreational supplies to self-mutilate; they used their newly acquired cosmetics to paint their scars.

We should note that, while token economies appear to be very simple system to develop and operate in most settings, in correctional institutions they are not simple by any means. In order to ensure that the correctional environment is managed in accord with operant principles, which is a necessity of behavioral programs, one must provide continuing surveillance and monitoring and be prepared to introduce change anywhere in the system at any time. Failure to do so may mean that the wrong behaviors are reinforced and maintained and that the staff are, in effect, working at cross-purposes to the program goals. Accordingly, when we expanded our program, we introduced a highly sophisticated token economy into an environment which had been prepared through staff training and modified management practices to function as an operant system.

The program incorporated sequential stages, or levels, through which each girl progressed as she earned her return to community living through the performance of specified behaviors. As she was promoted she enjoyed gradually increasing freedom, material comforts, and privileges, accompanied by increased responsibility for her own behavior. An extensive variety of reinforcers (such as weekend leaves, cosmetics, clothes, and community recreation programs) were provided throughout the program and were programmed such that their availability to any girl was a function of her stage placement. A girl, by earning promotion, could greatly improve her environment and increase her access to a variety of reinforcers as well as reduce the duration of her incarceration. Many of the privileges available in each stage were provided to a particular girl only as a function of her ability to purchase them through earned behavior credits. In addition to the token economy, individualized behavior contracts were utilized within each stage, whereby the girl, through performing specified behaviors, could earn certain privileges or commodities not ordinarily available in that stage. The amount of surveillance and the number of explicit contingencies varied from stage to stage such that there was a gradual transition from external control to self-control, both in terms of freedom from supervision and in terms of the relationship between privileges and behavior. Phasing out of behavior modification procedures was arranged during the final stage of the program in order to provide a gradual transition from the token economy to community life.

Prior to the introduction of the expanded program, considerable effort was expended in developing techniques of rating behavior which would be reliable and simple, which would be amenable to efficient recording and tabulation and would involve behaviors which were precisely defined and could be objectively recorded. Two lists of a large number of behaviors were obtained. The behaviors were those which were judged to be important to a girl's adjustment in the institution and in her postinstitutional environment and which also would lend themselves to precise and reliable recording. One list included prosocial acts (positive behaviors) which she ought to perform, while the other included antisocial or inappropriate acts (negative behaviors) which she would have to avoid if she were to cope adequately.

The girls' supervisors and teachers were instructed to observe and record the occurrence of a small number of these behaviors at any one rating period. The particular behaviors selected from the list for observation varied from time to time, and the girls were not informed as to which behaviors were being rated. Only the total list was made available to them.

The rating was conducted through a critical incident technique. Thus, each observed occurrence of the behavior was recorded and was summated at the end of each period to determine how many behavior credits had been earned. In this program a credit was earned if a girl emitted, in a particular period, more than a minimum of number of positive behaviors and fewer than a maximum of negative behaviors.

This rating system for negative behaviors, we must note, is similar to most of the behavior modification strategies employing an omission-checking system which records the nonoccurrence of specified behaviors. Such systems are used in many token economies and particularly in correctional settings.

Other contingencies, of course, were used as means of promoting adaptation to institutional demands. Thus, aversive consequences such as time out from reinforcement or loss of privileges were made contingent on major antisocial acts. We also employed extinction procedures, intermittent reinforcement schedules, and individualized behavior contracts (Ross and McKay, 1978b).

Each girl was assigned to a program adviser who, in addition to providing behavioral counseling, served as a kind of behavioral bank manager. They ensured that the girl was continually appraised of all aspects of the program on the basis of their observations of the girl's adjustment. The advisers also worked with the program coordinator, chief psychologist, interns, and consultants in providing staff training and supervision. Staff training was provided on a continuing basis throughout the treatment phases of our research. Extensive use was made of many audiovisual aids such as tape recordings of instructions which were available around the clock and videotaped demonstrations of the application of reinforcement techniques, behavior ratings, and the like. Weekly and, at times, daily small-group presentations were substituted for didactic presentations. Individual interviews were also arranged, again on a continuing basis, for all supervisors and teachers to ensure that they were aware of all aspects of the program and, particularly, to discuss the specific techniques to be used with individual cases. Representatives of the psychology service were available for information or consultation twenty-four-hours a day, seven days a week.

A manual describing every aspect of the program in complete detail was made available to every staff member and every girl. Lists of target behaviors, reinforcements, contingencies, rules, and consequences were posted throughout the institution and made available to all staff members and girls. The interaction of the supervisors and teachers with the girls was monitored in an effort to maximize the degree to which these interactions were in accord with behavior modification principles.

In all phases of the project, including the pilot studies, we employed several procedures in an attempt to ensure that appropriate behavior yielded approval by the group, in addition to the rewards provided in the economy. This was done in the hope that peer group reinforcement would become contingent on prosocial rather than antisocial acts. For example, special privileges were provided for all girls in a stage whenever any girl in that stage earned promotion. One of the target behaviors was "encouraging other girls to behave," and frequently, individual contracts were established whereby a girl could earn special rewards by attempting to improve the behavior of selected peers.

The operant program encompassed all of the girls' activities, including school, recreation, and residence life, for twenty-four hours a day throughout her stay in the institution. After her graduation, each girl was placed in the community and was on placement under the supervision of an after-care officer unttl her eighteenth birthday. An excellent adjustment to the community could lead to earlier termination of supervision.

We should note that in this program we used one other behavioral approach to the control of maladaptive behavior: extinction, that is, withholding reinforcement. According to the paradigm, behavior that is not reinforced will decrease in frequency. Assuming that carving represented attention-seeking or retaliatory behavior, we urged the staff to refrain from reinforcing it by giving undue attention to it through counseling, reprimanding, or discussing it with the girls. Instead, they were to automatically and without fuss impose the programatically determined consequences in a matter-of-fact manner. It became very clear that the staff simply could not follow our instructions in this instance. They were unable to avoid responding to the cuts on the girls' bodies and commented on them critically, were solicitous to the girl, or simply showed their revulsion by their facial expressions. We were convinced that extinction procedures (nonreinforcement) were not possible in the case of such behavior. Moreover, the other girls continued to provide considerable attention to this behavior. We were soon forced to drop extinction techniques.

Further descriptions of this program have been provided in other publications (Ross and McKay, 1975; 1976a,b, 1978). This program was a sophisticated, elaborate token economy which incorporated what were considered to be the best aspects of behavior modification techniques. It served as a model for programs which were introduced in many other institutions. It was far more impressive than that employed in the pilot behavior modification program which had been so successful. The only shortcoming of this new program was that it was a total failure.

The phase 1 behavior modification program led to a dramatic increase in the frequency of carving. During a six-month period 183 separate episodes of carving occurred in an experimental group of fifteen girls. In contrast, in a matched control group of fifteen girls who received only the standard training school program only 101 episodes of carving occurred.

The substantial increase in carving that was found in the phase 1 behavior modification program is, we hypothesize, a function of the inordinate concern with antisocial behavior that a negative rating system can engender. In an omission-checking system, privileges are contingent upon the absence of antisocial acts. We determined which negative behaviors had to be controlled for adequate ward management; we defined them precisely and carefully and explained to the correctional staff exactly what constituted the occurrence of an antisocial response (including carving). Our concern about the specification of such acts also implied the expectation that they would occur, and occur frequently enough to require constant surveillance. The supervisors came to perceive their role as lookouts for antisocial behavior. Each girl was given feedback on her behavior following specified intervals and was, therefore, reminded of all her antisocial acts. Our need to specify the behaviors also served to stimulate discussion among the staff and the girls as to the various forms which antisocial behavior could take.

Furthermore, the staff became hypervigilant in watching for antisocial acts and came to be perceived by the girls as watchdogs who should be avoided as much as possible since their presence was a discriminative stimulus for losing behavior credits. The girls may actually have been learning to avoid being observed and rated while committing antisocial acts. In other words, they were learning not to be caught. The supervisors reported frequently that they felt that "something was going on" but were unable to "catch them at it." The patients, then, came to be viewed very suspiciously by the staff. The supervisors were rewarded for their vigilance and found support for their suspicions in the profusion of concealed scars. Throughout the ward, in a vicious cycle, more and more emphasis came to be placed on carving and on applying programmed consequences to its occurrence.

It seems, then, that through an omission-checking system one can overrespond to antisocial behavior. We were attentive to it, we expected it, we advertised it, and we got it.

The consequence of our best behavioral programming efforts was to establish self-fulfilling prophecies for self-mutilation.

Need we mention another retreat to our offices?

The following summarizes our research sequence to this point:

1. traditional institutional remedies
2. carving study
3. intensive treatment milieu
4. pilot behavior modification program
5. phase 1 behavior modification program

Phase 2 Behavior Modification Program

Our interpretation of the discrepancy between the failure of the phase 1 program and the success of the pilot program led us to the development of an improved behavior modification program which was strictly positive in emphasis. The phase 2 behavior modification program differed from the phase 1 program in that rewards were now made contingent only upon performance of specified positive social acts. Behavior credits were earned for prosocial behavior regardless of whether the girls committed antisocial or inappropriate behaviors. Carving was not rated.

The results of the revised treatment program appear at first glance to be much more reassuring for the behavior modification enthusiasts. Fifteen experimental subjects in this treatment carved a total of 74 times in comparison with fifteen matched participants in the phase 1 program who had carved 183 times, and in comparison with fifteen matched participants in a no treatment control group who carved 101 times.

A positive approach can help. However, there were 74 instances of self-mutilation among the girls. We had not found a panacea. We certainly had not eliminated self-mutilation. Our riddle continues.

Complicating our lives is the following fact: In the positive program, the phase 2 behavior modification program, there was a considerable reduction in carving relative to the phase 1 program or the no treatment controls, but this was a reduction in the total number of carving episodes. There was not a reduction in the number of girls who carved themselves. In the traditional training school approach to prevent carving by punishment, in the no treatment controls, 66 percent of the girls carved on a total of 101 occasions. When extra emphasis was placed on negative consequences of carving the same percentage (66 percent) carved, but they did so much more frequently (181 episodes). When less emphasis was placed on carving in the positive phase 2 program, the frequency of carving was greatly reduced (74 episodes), but at least as many girls carved. In fact, 80 percent of the group mutilated themselves by carving!

Back to our offices.

Phase 2 Behavior Modification Plus Peer Therapist Program

One of the advantages of a behavioral approach to treatment is that it requires the therapist to keep careful records of his patients' behavior and ongoing environmental events. Our adoption of a behavioral approach to treatment and a sequential approach to research forced us to look back at the detailed behavioral data we had maintained throughout our research in order that we might explain the discrepancy between the extraordinary success of the pilot behavior modification program and the failure of the programs which had been developed from it. Reexamination of our research notes and behavioral data for the pilot program revealed that factors other than the behavior modification token economy may have been involved in our program. One of the girls in the program, Melinda (a pseudonym), had become enthused about the potency of behavior modification methodology in interpersonal manipulation and had learned enough about reinforcement techniques to apply them herself. Through the leadership of this bright, charming, delightfully manipulative offender, the girls had developed and were conducting a behavior modification program of their own. They were charting each other's behaviors, using explicit contingencies in their interactions, and even shaping the behavior of the staff!

We hypothesized that the success of our pilot program was attributable to the combination of this peer program and the token economy. We reasoned that improving the token economy used in the pilot program and maintaining the peer aspects might maximize the efficacy of our treatment even beyond the extraordinary success of our pilot program.

Consequently, in the next stage of our study (phase 2 behavior modification plus peer therapist program), the sophisticated (phase 2) positive behavior modification program used in the previous stage was maintained, but a new factor was added to the treatment approach: peer training. Girls in the token economy were provided with specific training in reinforcement therapy principles and encouraged to utilize these principles in attempting to modify the behavior of their peers.

Our results?

For matched groups of fifteen participants during six months of program the incidence of carving was: traditional training school no treatment controls: 101 episodes; phase 1 behavior modification program: 183 episodes; and phase 2 behavior modification program: 74 episodes. Our improved program incorporating the peer aspects led to 54 episodes of carving. In contrast to the pilot program, our new program reduced carving but it did not eliminate it. Sixty-six percent of the girls carved. That is the same number of girls who carved in the control group which received the traditional training school program.

We had come a long way, but we appeared to have made little progress. Where did we go wrong? Or more appropriately perhaps, where did we go right? Do not forget we said we eliminated carving three times. We have told you about one of those times—the pilot behavior modification program. We have told you what we did in that program. In the next chatper we will tell you what we later recognized that we had really done. We will also tell you about the other two times we eliminated self-mutilation at Grandview.

8 Co-opting

A Reappraisal

We were perplexed by the success of our pilot behavior modification program—a simplistic token economy—and the relative failure of our much more sophisticated token economies. Our sequential research strategy had led us to the development of an exemplary token economy program which served as a model for similar, even identical programs in other correctional institutions and in the adolescent units of several psychiatric hospitals. The program was exemplary in every way but its efficacy.

The phase 2 behavior modification plus peer therapist program had been developed on the basis of our reexamination of what we thought were important variables in our highly successful pilot program. In reexamining the pilot program we had concluded that the key to its success was the peer reinforcement aspects of the intervention. Faced with the failure of a program based on that interpretation, we not only reexamined the pilot operant program, we also reexamined the entire history of our work at Grandview. After all we had an obligation to our granting agency to explain why we were unable to replicate the success of a program which had shown such early promise and had stimulated the funding of our work. Not only did we reexamine the abundance of quantitative data that we had collected over the years, but also, for the first time, we seriously examined the qualitative data. Throughout the program we had kept diaries which chronicled in detail the life of the institution. We also had kept a running account of our personal impressions of the institutional atmosphere, the girls' perception of our programs, and the relationship between the staff and girls.

We even examined the original carving study. You will recall that in describing the carving study we told you that it was important. It was. We did not realize how important until some four years later when we reexamined our notes. It was important for none of the reasons you might imagine.

In the carving study we investigated carving by means of interviews, sociometric analysis, and personality testing. Would it surprise you to learn that, among the participants, after the study was underway and for a month and a half after it was over, self-mutilation ceased? Could such a simple little descriptive study lead to such a major change in the girl's behavior? If so, how?

We had paid little attention to the aftermath of the carving study because it never occurred to us that there would be one. We certainly did not expect a reduction in carving because of our research. We had not been interested in treating the behavior at that time; we were merely studying it.

Artifact? We thought so at first. We had been trained to treat correlation between apparently remote events with extreme caution. Initially, we gave very little thought to the decrease in carving, automatically attributing it to some vagary of the institutional life cycle, or to some temporary and insignificant lull in a fad, or to simple chance. In and of itself it may have had little significance, but taken together with the cessation of carving which occurred in the pilot program, a finding which we did not understand, it began to intrigue us.

We had eliminated carving twice. Once in the pilot program; the first time in the carving study. Could there be some connection between the first time and the second time? What similarity, we asked ourselves, was there in these apparently disparate events? What could the carving study and this treatment program possible have in common?

In reexamining our research notes we discovered factors which were operative in the carving study and the pilot program but absent in all the other treatment programs. The significance of these factors, how they might affect carving, began to dawn on us only after we looked again at what some of the girls had told us during the pilot program when we discussed their views of institutional living and their ideas as to what motivated girls to carve. When we put together what they told us with our conclusions as to the key ingredients in the carving study and the pilot program we radically altered our conceptualization of the motivational basis of carving. We also began to realize why the pilot program had been so successful and why the behavioral programs which it had stimulated had failed.

Autopsy of Success

There were at least two characteristics of the carving study and the pilot program which distinguished them from the other treatment programs. One was our unusual reaction to the girls' carving. The other was our unusual relationship to the girls.

In the carving study we spent a great deal of time talking with the girls. Our conversations were not limited to the structured interview conducted by our research staff. We had many conversations in which, frankly, we indulged our curiousity about the girls' self-mutilatory behavior. We were genuinely fascinated by their behavior. We wanted to learn as much as possible about how they carved, when they carved, and under what circumstances. We were interested in the mechanics of their cutting, the logistics, the techniques, the instruments, the designs, the antecedents, the attendant emotions at every stage of the process, the significance of the act for them, and the consequences. Our curiosity submerged our personal reactions to their behavior. We were behaving more like anthropologists that clinical psychologists; we were more interested in observing than diagnosing, evaluating, or judging. We were seeking the *how* more than the *why*.

We were told later by some of the girls that our attitude contrasted dramatically with their previous experience with professionals who had tried to stop them from carving or treated their behavior as pathological. We did not attempt to stop, prevent, control, or punish their behavior in any of the traditional ways. Moreover we clearly conveyed to the girls that we knew very little about their behavior or about what living in such a place was like. We openly and honestly admitted our naivete—a unique demeanor for institutional staff.

In talking with the girls, we treated them not as patients but as resource persons. They became active participants in our search for an understanding of the phenomenon. This was an information-sharing process distinctly different from therapeutically designed interactions. Through our conversations the girls became much more than simply our research subjects. They were now our research assistants! Our attitude reflected that they had become collaborators in our research.

The girls began to think we were so fascinated with their behavior that we were pleased when they carved—a development which would have alarmed the institution's director!

Could our unusually intense and persistent curiosity and our unorthodox approach to the girls somehow be related to the diminution of self-mutilation? It does not seem likely. If anything, it should increase carving. If carving is attention seeking, as is often thought, our attention would reinforce and augment the behavior. It did not. The behavior stopped. Why? We think that by our response to the girls and our attitude to carving we unwittingly robbed it of its instrumental value. Furthermore, we think we took the fun out of it. That interpretation occurred to us when we thought about our response to the girls' carving in the light of what some of them had told us about their perception of the reality of institutional life and the function that carving served for them.

Return to Melinda

One of the most persuasive and insightful of the many Grandview girls whom we came to depend upon as our unofficial research assistants was Melinda. You will remember Melinda, the charming adolescent girl who had started the girls' own behavior modification program. Melinda was a *wheel* in every sense of that term in institutional jargon. With her superior intelligence and manipulative skills, she effectively controlled the girls and subtly directed much of the staff's activities. She also had a fund of knowledge about the girls, the staff, the institution, and the intricacies of institutional life. Melinda told us a great deal about carving. To paraphrase her:

> It's my body and I can do anything I want with it. It's mine—it's the only thing I control completely. I'm its boss. The staff, the kids, or you

> and your rules can't stop me from doing anything if I want to do it. If I want to carve, I can—you can't stop me. If I want to get fat, I can. If I want to look ugly, I can. You guys can punish me—so what—I'm in control. If you punish me then I control you as well as me.

Melinda told us that by their carving the girls controlled what she called the "Grandview emergency machine." When the girls carved they started a chain reaction: the supervisors called in head supervisors; the head supervisor called the duty administrator; the administrator came running and summoned a retinue of professionals—the nurse, the doctor (if you cut deeply enough), the ambulance (if you really do it right), the caseworker, the male staff (if you are obstreperous about it or keep cutting instruments in view), and even the psychiatrist (if you threaten to keep doing it). Virtually guaranteed was a visit to the school's director. It was all so predictable.

Carving: A Reconceptualization

When we reexamined our notes on what Melinda and other girls had told us, we began to entertain an alternative conceptualization of the motivational basis of carving which might help us to understand how we had eliminated carving in the carving study and the pilot program through our unusual attitude to carving and our unorthodox relationship with the girls. We hypothesized that carving was the girls' way of expressing independence, autonomy, and personal freedom. It was a proprietary act. The girls perceived it as an expression of their freedom to do something they wanted to do. It was more than just a symbol of adolescent striving for independence or their way of opposing adult infringement on their personal freedom. It was a very elegant way of controlling their social environment. Through this behavior they could initiate and control adult intervention. By judiciously timing their carving, and by skillfully varying the depth of their cutting, the girls could determine when adult intervention would occur, what form it would likely take, and how intense it would be. The amount of adult attention could also be determined by the appropriate selection of the setting in which the girl carved. Some girls, we learned, could predict quite accurately how many staff members would be summoned; how quickly they would respond; how many stitches would be required; whether or not their parents would have to be notified; and how many interviews with their caseworker or psychologist would be forthcoming.

The attention that their behavior engendered was secondary to the feeling of power and control that carving achieved for them. They could obtain such feelings without experiencing the attention that carving typically produced. Merely knowing that they had such power gave them a sense of control over their lives, a feeling of satisfaction. It gave them enormous power. There was nothing we as adults could do about it—and that's fun.

> All I have to do to get the institution to jump is to put a little cut on my skin.

In a setting in which all of their daily activities were externally controlled, carving represented the ultimate in freedom, the epitome of personal freedom by which they could reassure themselves that they had some mastery over their fate.

It has been demonstrated that the loss of a feeling of personal control over one's life can engender vandalism (Zimbardo, 1970), school violence (National Institute of Education, 1978) and suicide (Lefcourt, 1976; Hatton, Valente, and Rink, 1977), and unexplained death for no apparent pathogenic cause (Lefcourt, 1976).

> To do a thing (or do in a thing) for its own sake is to show the arbritrariness of your personal power and the purely personal forces controlling the action. [Zimbardo, 1970, p. 8]

We do not wish to suggest that all forms of self-mutilation can be explained in terms of attempts to establish a feeling of personal control. It is merely a way of conceptualizing the carving behavior of our clients. However, some investigators have commented on the apparent controlling function of other forms of self-mutilation. Self-injurious behaviors have been viewed as means of controlling such things as fears of violence (Mintz, 1964), aggressive impulses (Mintz, 1964), sexual thoughts (Davidson, 1962), and social reinforcement (Foxx and Azrin, 1973; Morrison, 1972).

Cookson (1977) described self-mutilation among women prisoners as a reaction to feelings of helplessness. Burnham (1969) suggested that the mutilator "retires into self-sufficiency, beyond the reach of all who are involved with her" (p. 228). Rosenthal et al., (1972) described self-cutting as a response to an overwhelming event by an act which the patient can regulate. Similarly, Bach-Y-Rita (1974) described some self-mutilatory behavior as a response which substitutes for coping behavior that is blocked by externally imposed controls. Smolev (1971) suggested that self-injurious behavior controls the actions of other people through its aversive effects. Podvoll (1969) interpreted self-mutilation as designed to "test the limits of the community's control." More general comments have been made by Cox and Klinge (1976) and Ferrence and Johnson (1974). Self-mutilators are seen as exercising control over an environment in which they have limited power.

There is a striking similarity between Melinda's comments to us and the following statement by a patient of Podvol (1969) who, after she had cut her arms said:

> These are my arms; I do with them as I please, whenever I please. If I choose to make them ugly, they will be ugly. [P. 220]

It is also interesting to note Gold and Coghlan's (1975-76) study. They found that, as measured by Rotter's locus of control (I–E) scale, self-mutilating female drug users tended to believe that their lives were controlled by "luck, fate, chance, or more powerful others," that is, their locus of control was more external than that of nonmutilators. It has also been reported that schizophrenic children who were able to verbalize (and, presumably, better able to control their environment) mutilated less than nonverbal schizophrenics (Shodell and Reiter, 1968).

The foregoing explanations provide some support for our conceptualization. However, the investigators who refer to the controlling function of self-mutilation typically deemphasize its explanatory power, tending to include it as one of a number of explanations and to give preference to conceptualizations in terms of psychopathology. With the exception of the behaviorally oriented investigators, most suggest treating the underlying psychopathology rather than dealing directly with the controlling function of the behavior.

Prescription for Failure

If our reconceptualization of the motivational basis of carving is valid, it is clear why our behavioral programs failed to eliminate carving. These programs were the epitome of adult-inspired and externally imposed programs which unabashedly attempted to control every aspect of the adolescents' lives. At the best of times this institution severely restricted the girls' freedom. The sophisticated phase 1 behavioral program, which sensitized the staff to negative behaviors and explicitly punished carving, reduced the girls' degrees of freedom to zero. By so doing we effectively, though inadvertedly, augmented the use of carving as a means of enabling the girls to perceive that they had some control over their lives and us.

Programs which explicitly punish or treat carving proclaim that carving is something only the girls want to do and reinforce their view that they are acting independently when they do carve. The behavior modification plus peer therapist program provided them with an alternative means of perceiving that they had some control, but it too was imposed by us, and the girls came to see it as just another way of our controlling them. They still had a reason to carve.

Prescription for Success

We concluded that there were two key factors contributing to the elimination of carving in the pilot program and in the carving study.

First, our attitude to the girls' carving, our obviously genuine curiosity and fascination, was perceived by them as inconsistent with the typical staff reaction of abhorrence or condemnation. Our reaction reflected interest, not disapproval. Because of our strong interest as researchers, they began to think that we were getting something out of it—a personal benefit. They questioned whether they were carving for themselves or for us. How could they control us by an oppositional behavior which we did not oppose? How could they proclaim their autonomy through this behavior unless we proclaimed that we did not want them to do it? They decided to stop entertaining us.

Second, by relating to the girls as adjunct research staff we placed them in a therapeutic bind. How, when acting as competent, intact, intelligent research associates could they continue to do "a dumb thing like carving"?

Moratorium on Treatment

Obviously the foregoing explanations are decidedly post hoc. No doubt alternative and equally plausible explanations could be posited. We viewed them as interesting hypotheses which formed the basis for our final treatment program in which we tested an intervention strategy which eliminated self-mutilation in Grandview for the third time.

We refer to our strategy as *co-opting*. It entails persuading the girls that by carving they are cooperating with those whose control they oppose.

To establish the groundwork for co-opting, we terminated all behavior modification and other formalized treatment programs in the institution. We gave up the appearance of control in order that we could establish the basis for gaining real control over the girls' carving.

Co-opting Carving

If the girls believed that carving was something that we did not really oppose, carving would not serve its purpose of giving them a feeling of personal control. How could we persuade the girls that their self-mutilation was a behavior of which we did not disapprove when we really wished that they would stop it? We could not just say, "I want you to carve." To do so would be unethical, perhaps illegal. Furthermore, the girls would not belive us and would immediagely test the validity of the statement by carving even more.

Our approach was much more subtle. It was a multifaceted strategy designed to convince the girls that they could no longer view carving as a proprietary act or a declaration of independence.

Curiosity

We systematically reestablished the kind of relationship we had achieved with the girls during the carving study and the pilot program. As in those programs, because of our apparent fascination, the girls came to question whether by continuing to carve they would be serving their needs for control or our investment in their behavior; whether they were carving for us or for themselves.

In the carving study this expression of curiosity was spontaneous and genuine. In the new program our curiosity was planned and deliberate. There was a risk that our response would appear contrived. Accordingly, we felt we could not rely solely on our planned curiosity. We added two other elements in our attempts to convince the girls that carving could not serve its purpose.

De-pathologizing

Behavior can be controlled to some extent by the labels which are assigned to it. For example, ear piercing and tattooing are really self-mutilatory, but we call them decorative. Elective surgery is self-mutilatory, but we call it therapeutic. Self-mutilatory behavior in many cultures is socially approved, even required as a rite de passage–it is socially appropriate. By calling behaviors positive or prosocial or adaptive, we encourage and foster them. At least this is so in the case of individuals who choose to accept our frame of reference, who share our values. But in the instance of carving, these adolescents were behaving in opposition to our values. When we behaved as though carving was pathological, grotesque, or abnormal, we made it clear to the girls that we wanted them not to do it. By doing it they asserted their independence from us. They felt in control.

In most institutions there are antagonistic forces working in opposition to one another–inmates and staff. They see things from radically different points of view. What would happen if the warring parties adopted the other's point of view? What if, at Grandview, we stopped viewing carving as pathological or even problematic; What if we stopped responding to it as behavior designed to attack the staff's power or values and saw it as the girls perceived it to be–a genuine attempt to cope with an excessively controlling environment?

What if we then stopped opposing it and talked about it as consistent with the staff's values? What if we next relabeled their self-mutilation and responded to it not as oppositional but as compliant behavior which testifies that they are complying with the principles apparently underlying the environment we have created? After all, we proclaimed that we wished to promote the emotional development of these adolescents. We wished them to begin acting as mature individuals. But autonomy and independence are the hallmarks of maturity. If the girls came to perceive carving as a sign that they were developing maturity, by carving they would be collaborating with us, yielding to our control.

We relabeled carving. We responded to it as a creative act–epidermal art–an act of independence and maturity. By so doing we took the fun out of it.

De-romanticizing

Our open relationship with the girls allowed them to tell us about their perception of institutional life and the role that carving played for them. The relationship also allowed us to tell them about our own perception of their environment. The girls thought that by carving they were exercising their independence by refusing blatantly and dramatically to accept the explicit demands of the institution for good behavior. Our view was that by doing so they were indeed satisfying the implicit needs of the staff by imbuing their otherwise dull institutional lives with some meaning and purpose. Job satisfaction for institutional employees is often based on the stimulation generated by inmates' behavior. Only if the girls misbehaved could the staff feel they were needed.

We were able to admit to the girls that crises were exciting. In the past the girls had told us that escaping was fun. What we had not been able to admit was that searching for them was even more fun. Our professional roles had forced us to adopt a very serious demeanor and to chastise the girls for conduct which most of the staff secretly enjoyed. Crisis intervention may be serious, but it is also exciting. The activities involved for the staff are precisely those that the girls could view as fun if they were doing them. They had little trouble understanding that their carving might serve to provide the staff with stimulation.

No matter how persuasive we might have been, the girls could not completely accept our arguments on the basis of logic alone. Even the girls believed in hypothesis testing. They stopped carving and discovered a new game. Whereas their carving had engendered excitement, their failure to carve engendered suspicion. The staff felt "they were up to something" and went to great lengths to discover what it was. Viewing the girls' cessation of carving as a "lull before the storm," the institutional machinery was now set for imminent disturbance. The girls began to believe that the staff would breathe a collective sign of relief if they carved!

This was a new experience for the girls and served to entrench the tentative conclusions to which they were being led by our fascination with their behavior. The staff were getting as much, if not more, out of their behavior than they were. They then became convinced that they could better proclaim their autonomy by refusing to carve, which they did. They came to oppose carving with almost as much vehemence as we had demonstrated in our treatment programs.

Co-opting the Girls

The cessation of carving among the girls in the carving study continued for a month and a half after the study was completed. In the pilot program the elimination of carving was maintained throughout the remainder of the girls' stay in the institution, a period of four months. We believe that we can attribute the cessation of carving in the pilot program to the same factors we previously indicated as responsible for this effect in the carving study. An additonal factor, we believe, was responsible for the persistence of this effect in the pilot program. The girls found an alternative means of obtaining a feeling that they had some control over their environment.

The cessation of carving occurred because through our interest in carving the girls became our resident experts for whom continuing to carve would be incompatible with their new image of themselves. When our interests declined at the end of the study, there was no reason for them not to resume carving since they no longer were being treated as experts. However, in the pilot program, by means of a simple but elegant resolution, they were able to maintain the feeling of expertise without returning to carving. They became therapists. Like ex-addicts in self-help groups for alcoholism, they became *professional ex-carvers* dedicated to stamping out carving through their behavior modification program. Thereby, they obtained a feeling that they were controlling their environment by means of prosocial behavior which was consistent with their new image as paraprofessionals.

In order to ensure that the cessation of carving would not be merely temporary, we determined that we should persuade the girls to learn a new means of coping with their environment. We set out to convince them that they could control their environment much more effectively by means of prosocial behavior.

We were quite confident that we could convince the girls that they could control their environment because our experience had convinced us that they always had controlled it! The control of the institution which correctional staff often think that they have is, in actuality, very limited. Economic, social, and political forces outside the correctional institution often are the powers by which it is regulated. However, the actual control of the correctional environment is determined, not by the politics of the society at large, but by the dictates of the society within, the inmate society. The inmate's strategies for controlling themselves and the staff are much more powerful than any officially sanctioned program. They run the show (Ross and Price, 1976).

In effect the girls already had considerable control over the environment, and we did not have to convince them that they did. However, their control was oppositional and antagonistic to the values and goals prescribed by the institution. They promoted antisocial behavior through their counterculture. We wished to use their power to work for us rather than against us.

The power in the institution was not, of course, shared equitably by all the girls. In any inmate subculture most of the power lies in the hands of an elite group—the wheels. Each unit at Grandview had its "Godmother" who commanded a "family" of eager subordinates who at her direction dispensed the real rewards and punishments in the institution. They were the powerbrokers who unofficially managed the institution. Recognizing this, we determined that the way to correct the inmate culture was to *turn the wheels*.

Turning the Wheel

We already had some experience in converting a wheel from a leader who promoted antisocial behavior to one who directed a group of girls toward prosocial behavior. Melinda had, through the peer group behavior modification program she managed, mobilized her peer group into an impressive force promoting prosocial behavior. However, what had occurred with Melinda had developed spontaneously and naturally. We had not asked her to do it. We were surprised when we discovered she had done it. It was her idea, not something she was doing at our urging. How with the new group of girls in our final treatment program could we motivate their wheel to run a similar program?

If we asked the new leader to establish a new program she would likely reject the idea as merely another of our devices to control her. How could we have her run our program and yet feel that it was hers—something she was doing for herself, not for us? We wanted the girls to initiate a program on their own volition. We wanted them to promote prosocial behavior using behavioral techniques to control each other. Prosocial behavior and control: two concepts which were anathema to the girls.

The first component of our co-opting strategy—co-opting carving—converts the girls from research subjects to research assistants. The second component—co-opting the girls—converts a wheel into a therapist and then into a program director who manages a cadre of adolescent therapists.

Although we shall describe co-opting as a strategy with programmatic features, it should be realized that our agenda was at no time revealed to the girls. Although our plans were very carefully developed prior to implementation, we could not let it appear that the program was either conceived or initiated by adults or externally imposed.

Rascal to Client

The first wheel we attempted to convert in our new program was Debbie L., the girl whose case was presented in the prologue.

Debbie had a long history of self-mutilatory behavior. A wide variety of institutional placements and therapeutic interventions had failed to ameliorate her self-destructive behavior. In part because of her extensive institutional experience, in part because of her sophistication in delinquent activities, and in part because of her exceptional skills in interpersonal manipulation, Debbie became a leader of a large group of girls at Grandview. At first she gained the respect of the girls through her institutional know-how and her ability to manipulate both staff and girls into giving her what she wanted. She also was the "jail-house lawyer" on whom they came to depend to fight their battles with the staff. She gained their respect and admiration and became their champion. She acquired a retinue of followers eager to be accepted by her. She was their model and their master. Interestingly, as her renown increased, her self-mutilation decreased. Perhaps she did not need to carve in order to have a feeling of personal control; she had supreme control as the wheel. Debbie's other antisocial behavior also decreased. She was seldom personally involved in antisocial activities. However, consistent with her role as leader of the loyal opposition, she continually encouraged such behavior in her peers. Like Fagan in *Oliver Twist*, she commanded a group of apprentices whom she instigated, manipulated, and, at times, ordered to oppose the staff through various antisocial activities, including carving.

We set out to convert Debbie from a wheel devoted to promoting antisocial behavior in opposition to the staff to a leader who advocated prosocial behavior —a formidable task.

Client to Assistant

When we first invited Debbie L. to come for interviews with us she agreed to do so without hesitation. She was an old hand at using visits to the psychologist for secondary gain. An interview with the "shrink" represented an hour out of school, if nothing else.

We presented no threat to her. At Grandview, visiting the professionals even on a frequent basis bore no stigma. It was a practice which the girls promoted. Since the professionals spent most of their time interviewing girls after crises, one's status in the oppositional culture was measured by the amount of interview time one acquired. Debbie was able to maintain and even fortify her image as wheel by associating with the professional wheels. To the girls she could present her interviews with us in terms of her manipulating the institution. She took credit for many of the changes which we had promoted. Very soon in our interview schedule she decided to establish an affiliation with us.

Her decision to affiliate was motivated not only by her desire to enlist our power to bolster her own but also by basic human needs for recognition, acceptance, and approval. Even wheels get lonely. After all she was first and foremost an adolescent. As a wheel she had a relationship with her peers, but this was of necessity limited by her need to maintain distance appropriate to a position of authority and superior-subordinate relationships. Nor could she have a genuine close relationship with the matrons and at the same time maintain her position as leader of the opposition. We afforded Debbie the possibility of gaining the recognition and acceptance she needed but which she could never enjoy with her subordinates, and we enabled her to enter a relationship without jeopardizing her position in the inmate culture.

Our interviews also represented novelty for Debbie. She had been accustomed to being treated as a major problem in the institution—an undersocialized, manipualtive sociopath with a remarkable potential for mischief who, for purely personal gain, led the other girls into difficulty without concern for their welfare. She was seen as an untrustworthy, egocentric, callous, antisocial adolescent with many emotional problems. Her power over her peers was viewed as pathological. Such an assessment was not incompatible with her history.

Our response to Debbie was radically different. We quite explicitly denied her psychopathology. Our discussions dwelt exclusively on her personal strengths. Behavioral characteristics which had been couched in negative terms we relabeled in positive terms. We referred to her manipulativeness as social skill, her unreliability as flexibility, her domineering as leadership, her histrionics as creativity, her callousness as pragmatism, her suspiciousness as insight.

Without stretching credibility too far, we complimented, even flattered, her on any trait that was even remotely positive and exaggerated the importance of relatively insignificant prosocial acts. In short, we treated her as a competent individual rather than a problem-ridden patient. We responded to this antisocial wheel as a concerned, essentially altruistic, socially aware adolescent who was, through her leadership, helping the girls to adapt to an oppressive environment.

Debbie would not have accepted our treatment of her if it were not for the fact that we were sincere. She really was an unusually enterprising girl with outstanding interpersonal skills. The fact that she opposed all that we held dear in terms of good institutional adjustment should not detract from her outstanding leadership abilities. She was far better able to relate to the girls than we were, more able to understand them and to control them. In a way we had the same aims: to control the girls and to make them behave in accordance with our wishes. We could not really fault her on her motives.

We differed in two ways: our goals—she prescribed antisocial behavior, we prescribed prosocial behavior; our methods—hers worked, ours did not.

We came to respect Debbie's perception and insight. We had no difficulty in avoiding being judgmental about her behavior and were able to relate to her at all times in a positive manner.

Our relationship with Debbie had many of the essential ingredients of effective psychotherapy (empathy, warmth, unconditional positive regard), but it was by no means psychotherapy in the usual sense. We spent very little time discussing Debbie's personal concerns. We spent most of the time gaining information. This was not a typical client-therapist interaction. It was more of a teacher-student relationship. The psychologist was the student. Where other girls had been our research assistants who helped us understand institution life, Debbie was our visiting professor, assisting us in understanding her milieu. Debbie became our barometer of the institutional atmosphere and our sounding board for many decisions. We did these things very deliberately not only because we genuinely respected her knowledge but also because we wanted to alter her perception of her institutional role. Debbie began to see herself in a new light: not as an adversary of the professionals who directed programs that controlled her, but as our guru.

Assistant to Collaborator

The next step in our conversion of Debbie was to persuade her to cooperate with us in some aspects of our work. We wanted to have her begin acting like a therapist. But that represented a major role change. It was one thing to sit in an office and instruct us on institutional reality. It was another thing altogether to take an active part in our work. She had her self-respect and her image with the group to protect. She could not allow herself to be seen joining the enemy. Helping us would make her appear to be a turncoat and compromise her position as wheel. However, we were treating her as an altruistic person deeply concerned for the welfare of other girls, and she felt obliged to live up to this pleasant new image. We asked for her help, but made it easy for her to collaborate with us. Specifically, we told her about the difficulties we were having with some particularly problematic girls in another unit. We asked her to visit the other unit, make some observations, and give us an assessment of the girls which might help us understand how best to treat them. She could do this without her own group questioning her loyalty. When she cooperated with us, we responded to her as a junior psychologist, a diagnostician whose appraisal of a problem merited our most careful attention. She now was our cohort, and we treated her as a regular member of our staff. We involved her in many of our professional activities. She joined us in meetings in which we discussed various therapeutic approaches we might introduce to deal with those girls; she accompanied us to the university to read books and articles on the treatment of recalcitrant adolescents; she took professional visitors on tours of the institution and explained the philosophy and program of the psychology department; she even helped us train the doctoral candidates who were interning at Grandview!

Collaborator to Private Practitioner

Although we treated Debbie as one of our staff, we studiously avoided giving her any responsibility for treatment. We gave her tasks in public relations, in teaching our staff, and in assessing our clients, but never even suggested that she treat her peers. Nothing we asked of her threatened her power position with the girls. Her role as our adviser, our cohort, was perceived differently by her peers. They were convinced, with a little help from her, that she had us "wrapped around her little finger." Her status in the inmate group was elevated considerably through what appeared to be her brilliant manipulation of the authorities.

The next step Debbie took on her own accord. Debbie, like many other wheels whom we co-opted, was ambitious and eager for power. Cast in a role as junior psychologist, she was in a lesser position than some of her professional colleagues. Particularly irritating to her was her ranking below the interns, many of whom were not much older than she. They were part of our treatment team. She was not. Debbie knew only too well that we were not very successful in treating the girls' problems. She was confident that she could do so more successfully than us. In spite of our recognition of her talents we seemed to her to be denying her promotion from assistant to therapist. Through her reading, her attendance at meetings, her participation in the intern-training programs, she had acquired a sound understanding of our techniques, particularly our behavioral techniques. Like her predecessor, Melinda, she established her own therapy program for some of the girls in her group whose behavior was irritating to both her and her friends and was, incidentally, also distressing to us. She, then, in a delightfully nonchalant fashion, demonstrated to us the ease with which she brought the girls' behavior problems under control with our techniques.

We were, of course, delighted, not merely because she had ameliorated some behavior problems in our clients, but primarily because she had appointed herself as a therapist. She had begun behaving like us. She had, at least, temporarily, adopted our goals and our techniques as her own. She felt she had taken over control of our treatment efforts. She thought she had co-opted us. We thought we had co-opted her. Actually, we were co-operating.

Private Practitioner to Program Director

Debbie enjoyed her new role. Like any new therapist, she wanted to treat everybody. But she had a problem. She recognized that if she tried to treat her peers as patients she would have to forfeit her role as wheel. She also realized that unless she was a wheel her attempts to treat her peers would be rejected. She knew she could not be effective without the support of the inmate group. She was in a position identical to the one we ourselves had been in.

How could she be a wheel and at the same time be a therapist? We helped Debbie realize that there was only one way. She could be a wheel and a therapist if she convinced her peers to be therapists. She had to convert her peers. She also had to sever her connections with us in order to make sure the girls did not think she was simply a puppet. But she did so only temporarily. She reinstated her position with us after she had persuaded the girls to join her in her new enterprise. She obtained too much acceptance and recognition from us to be satisfied with the prestige of being a leader among the girls. Moreover, she was going to run the treatment program, and she did not want to miss our admiration for her success.

Debbie's conversion of her peers was far more efficient and straightforward than our conversion of her. She manipulated them into working for her in return for various concrete rewards and for her support and friendship (and probably her protection). She selected several close friends and allowed them to be her assistants. She trained them in simple reinforcement principles and persuaded them to use these with other less popular girls whose behavior was creating problems for the staff and leading to withdrawal of privileges in the unit. She also persuaded them to use behavioral techniques to modify the behavior of the staff!

After Debbie had established her program she reestablished her relationship with the psychology department and frequently brought with her to our meetings several of her *junior therapists*. We helped Debbie establish a managerial scheme for her program which incorporated several levels of therapists and program managers. When a new girl first entered the unit, she became the client of the peer therapist group. A case manager (one step up from a therapist) supervised her program. After several weeks of appropriate behavior the girl earned the privilege of being a student therapist and began a two-to-three-week training period under the tutelage of her former case manager. She was trained in the principles of behavior modification through lectures, demonstrations, films, and reading materials and given practice assignments in applying the techniques to selected new girls. On matriculation she became a practicing therapist. Exceptional achievements as a therapist could lead to her being appointed by Debbie as a program manager. Debbie, of course, was the program director. The program managers were selected partly on the basis of their potential as replacements for program director after Debbie's release from the institution. These were the girls who, under normal circumstances, would have become wheels.

Throughout the co-opting program not one incident of carving occurred among the girls who acted as therapists. In addition, in most cases, the number of institutional offenses (assault, property damage, and abscondance) became zero after the girls received a few weeks of training as therapists, and this improvement was maintained throughout their stay in the institution (Ross and McKay, 1976a,b; 1978b).

Principles of Co-opting

Clearly, co-opting is a multifaceted intervention approach encompassing many treatment techniques, some of which are similar to aspects of other treatment modalities. Our research did not allow us to determine which of the many factors involved, if any, were crucial. We tend to feel that all of them were important. However, in our view the following characteristics seem particularly significant.

Client's Perspective

Co-opting was developed not on the basis of any preconceived or fixed theoretical explanation of our clients' behavior problems. Rather than forcing our personal frame of reference on the girls' behavior, we allowed our conceptualization of the motivational basis of their behavior to develop from understanding our clients' view of their environment. Doing so led us to perceive the meaning of their behavior in terms clearly different from those suggested to us by our training and our reading of the literature. It also led us to a radical departure from traditional approaches to the treatment of self-mutilation.

Normalizing

In co-opting we studiously avoided the possibility that our behavior as therapists might have iatrogenic effects. We particularly avoided talking about our clients' behavior in pathological terms or in terms of personal deficiencies. We thereby avoided the labeling process that can maintain or even engender problematic behavior. In this regard we were guided not so much by the work of Szasz (1961), and Laing and Esterson (1964), or Glasser (1965) as by the work of Rosenthal and Jacobson (1968), Stuart (1970), and others who have argued that labels can create self-fulfilling prophecies. We quite explicitly denied our clients' pathology and focused instead on their competence, prosocial skills, and personal strengths, no matter how limited. We treated them as cohorts rather than clients; as therapists rather than patients. In effect we reversed the potentially pathology-engendering effect of diagnostic labeling and, instead, generated expectancies that our clients would behave as altruistic, prosocial, and capable individuals rather than as problem-ridden patients.

Power of the Peers

Co-opting clearly recognizes the role of social factors in engendering and maintaining problematic behavior and provides a mechanism to neutralize their effects. It provides a powerful means of mobilizing group pressure as a therapeutic force. We feel that such a process could be useful with many patient groups, but particularly with adolescents. In contrast to many programs in which adolescents feel they are coerced into changing their behavior by treatment imposed on them by adult authority figures, they see this program as their own. The professionals can remain as the out-group which the adolescents can oppose by taking over their program. They can co-opt adults.

Moreover, the adolescents see themselves as responsible for any changes in their behavior. Such self-attribution has been shown to be essential for the persistence of behavior change (Shaver, 1975).

Crabtree and Grossman (1974) achieved a major decrease in self-mutilatory behavior in their hospitalized adolescent psychiatric patients. They attributed their success to the establishment of a "wholesome community" with an "atmosphere of trust and good feeling," and to the establishment of "administrative clarity" and of an "open door policy" which gave responsibility (and respect) to their patients. In discussing their success they note that they mobilized "patients and staff to work more closely with high-risk patients." Regrettably, they did not describe the specific techniques they employed to "persuade" their patients to help other patients.

The peer therapist aspect of co-opting differs in several fundamental ways from other programs which employ patients as psychotherapeutic agents for each other. Many programs (for example, Alcoholics Anonymous, Synanon, Therapeutic Community, Positive Peer Culture) promote group confrontation and criticism as a major therapeutic mechanism. Group sanctions for nonconforming behavior are also common in some of these approaches. Such processes can lower self-esteem and are totally incompatible with the tenets of co-opting, which deals exclusively with personal strengths rather than with personal weaknesses.

Co-opting is not problem focused. Our clients are encouraged only toward positive and supportive interactions (positive reinforcement) with their peers. The peers clearly articulate to each other that punishment, censure, and negative confrontation are incompatible with their role as therapists. Any therapist who uses these techniques is likely to find herself as a patient of her peer therapists.

Finally in co-opting we require our clients to assume responsibility for their peers but we are not content to leave them to their own devices. We allow them to assume the responsibility but give them no formal authority except by way of calling them therapists. More important, we have an obligation to ensure that they are equipped to assume therapeutic responsibility. Accordingly, unlike some therapeutic community approaches, we provide our clients with formal training in a specific therapeutic technique. One of our clinical colleagues who recommended treating an impotent male and helping a frigid female by making them therapists for each other did not go far enough. We believe it is our responsibility to tell them how to do it!

Helper-Therapy Principle

The remarkable improvement which we observed in the behavior of our clients and in their self-esteem may be attributable to the "Helper" Therapy Principle, which suggests that therapy is often more beneficial to the helper than to the helpee (Reissman, 1965). We led the girls to believe, "I must be worthwhile if I can help others."

Before she was proclaimed as a "therapist" each girl was the client of other girls who had been in the institution longer and had been trained as "therapists". Our data show quite clearly that it was immediately after she became a "therapist" that a girl's adjustment improved markedly. Merely mobilizing her peer group to bring pressure to bear on an adolescent may be a necessary but insufficient strategy for engendering behavior change in that adolescent.

Relationship with Clients

Fundamental to co-opting is the establishment of a close relationship with the leaders of the client group. As Egan (1975) has pointed out, in any form of therapeutic intervention, it is essential that the therapist first establish an influence base with his client.

We feel that such a relationship was essential to the success of our program but doubt that it was sufficient. In co-opting we do not attempt to form a relationship with all of our clients; only with their leaders. We have very limited contact with most of the clients. To do otherwise would be to take over from the program leaders. The contact with most of our Grandview clients for other than routine administrative duties was restricted to assessment interview to provide consultation for the peer therapists; officiating at formal ceremonies to proclaim their promotion within the peer therapist *career ladder*; and infrequent discussions with them in which we co-opted self-mutilatory behavior. The latter sessions were very brief and entailed only one or two interviews in most cases.

Adolescent Advocates

Finally, co-opting provides a subtle but effective technique for modifying the client's self-perception. By treating our adolescents as advocates of prosocial behavior and by skillfully persuading them to encourage and reinforce prosocial behavior in their peers, we succeeded in having these adolescents become committed to prosocial attitudes and behavior themselves.

Co-opting translates into therapeutic practice Bem's (1967) theory of self-perception, which argues that one can become committed to a position through advocating it.

Postscripts and Cautionary Notes

Carving was only one of a large number of major behavior problems which we faced at Grandview. These girls had many chronic behavior problems which were intractable to many remedies. Carving was the most dramatic, and potentially damaging, of these behaviors. We have described our work with carving. Co-opting was equally successful with other self-mutilatory behaviors. Swallowing foreign objects, inserting needles and pins in their skin, tattooing, consuming toxic substances, deliberate falling, and other self-injurious behaviors had, like carving, been only too common in the institution. They ceased in our co-opting program. As noted previously, co-opting also led to the almost complete cessation of other serious misbehaviors including assault, abscondance, theft, and infraction of institutional rules. Vandalism, a perennial problem at the institution, was eliminated among the co-opting participants.

We have also given considerable thought to how co-opting might be applied to indirect self-injurious behaviors such as smoking, alcoholism, and obesity, and to other antisocial behaviors such as shoplifting and vandalism. But much caution has to be exercised before we attempt to extrapolate to new problems.

It is unfashionable for proponents of new therapeutic modalities to suggest that there are shortcomings in their technique. Too often, advocates, writing with missionary zeal, describe their approach as a new panacea which therapists, eager for new remedies, too readily adopt. We wish to present some precautionary notes for anyone who might consider trying co-opting. The cautions derive from the experience we had in our work at Grandview.

Some five months after it started, we were forced to terminate the co-opting program. It was successful, but perhaps, too successful.

One of the advantages of such a program is that it is very cost-efficient. Its operation requires very few professionals. The girls run the program, and they do not require the expertise of a large number of professionals. Adolescent therapists are needed; professional therapists are not. Such a program is not likely to be popular with professional staff. It certainly was not at Grandview.

Another factor which detracted in no small way from the popularity of co-opting was its explicit rejection of pathology in the clients. Such a notion could not be accepted by many of our colleagues in spite of the obvious failure of programs based on notions of psychopathology or personal deficiency. Some of our colleagues tried to drop their pathology biases and stop responding to the girls as inadequate, emotionally disturbed, and antisocial individuals, but their training or their job demands made their efforts both artificial and short-lived. We cannot fault them for this since we also found it extremely difficult to refrain from regressing to our former proclivity for pathology seeking. Perhaps they were unable to give up the romanticized perception of their work and the importance of their clinical expertise in dealing with disturbed adolescents.

Co-opting also required that they take a one-down position in their interactions with their clients and authentically present themselves as dependent on their clients' help. Most of our colleagues were as reluctant to relinquish the comfort of their established clinical oreintations and roles as they were to relinquish their jobs.

Our professional colleagues were joined by the institutional administrators when they voiced their concern that we were giving the girls too much power. These were disturbed adolescents who had to be controlled. Giving power to such girls was totally abhorrent in spite of the fact that it was clear that the girls were applying their power for prosocial purposes and were controlling each other far more effectively than they could be controlled by the staff. Moreover, we gave them no power which they did not already have in abundnace. We simple redirected it to be used in cooperation with us rather than in opposition to us.

We gave the girls responsibility, not authority. As several staff learned to their dismay when they subsequently tried to replicate what they thought was involved in our program, the peer aspects of co-opting do not entail giving the inmate group control over anything that they do not already control. We merely help them to develop an illusion of control. It is the staff who gain in terms of increased control; not the clients. At no time did we let the girls think they would be given any authority in any institutional activity. We made no promises that they would have any power in decision making. We did not make such promises because we knew we could not keep them. Staff who later led their girls to form student governments, councils, and representatives learned bitterly that such efforts only formalized the adversarial role of the inmate culture and increased the girls oppositional motivation by falsely promising them that they would have a say in the running of the institution.

Some of the clinical staff objected to our expressing interest in the girls' carving. They felt that such a response rewarded the girls for self-injurious behavior and constituted secondary gain. Some staff were so wedded to their perception that they could not accept the fact that the girls stopped carving when we responded in this fashion. Ironically, many of the same staff had totally rejected our earlier attempts to extinguish carving by withholding their attention when carving occurred!

Much more distressing for us were the clinicians who thought we were deliberately encouraging the girls to injure themselves. They made it clear to us that such behavior is reprehensible. We totally agree. Or at least we would if we had really done what they thought we were doing. They were wrong on two counts. First, the results of our response to the girls' carving make it clear that it had the effect of discouraging rather than encouraging their self-mutilatory behavior. Second, at no time did we actively encourage the girls to carve. Rather we very deliberately and quite openly refused to discourage carving. Conceptually and ethically there is a fine line between failing to discourage and actively encouraging. Anyone who wishes to use co-opting with any problematic behavior must take great care to ensure that they or their clients do not confuse the two.

In co-opting we do not attempt to have the patient practice his sympton as is the case in negative practice (Dunlap, 1932) and paradoxical intentionality training (Frankl, 1960). There may well be commonalities in the theoretical rationale of such therapies and of co-opting, but not in terms of technique. As we noted earlier, to have encouraged or pretended to encourage any of our adolescent patients to carve would have been to invite a bloodbath. They would have immediately recognized that we were just manipulating them, trying to trick them into stopping, which would have signified even more clearly to them that we wanted them to stop. The girls were not dull.

We made it clear that we were not trying to stop them from doing it. We did not communicate this explicitly because they would not have believed our statement. We did so by expressing our genuine interest, which they took to mean that we were not opposed to their behavior. Our decision to respond in this way was not taken lightly. We were convinced by our considerable experience with these girls that our response would be interpreted by them in just that way and *not* as our urging them to carve. We also made a careful assessment of each case. The application of co-opting to other behaviors and other clients must include a very careful assessment of the clients' interpretation of the therapist's intent.

Ironically, many of the staff who expressed their feelings that we were encouraging self-mutilation did not take the same view of their punishment techniques which actually did encourage the girls' self-mutilatory behavior. We were adamant in our refusal to support the staff in their desire to punish carving. Our colleagues frequently reminded us of the work of Lovaas who used punishment effectively in controlling the self-injurious behavior of patients. Without raising debate as to the ethical issues involved in aversive conditioning, we should point out that such techniques held little promise for controlling the carving behavior of our clients. Carving did not occur with the high frequency that characterizes the head banging or self-slapping behavior that has been treated by aversive conditioning. Judging by the number of trials that are required to eliminate such repetitive behaviors our patients would have had to carve and be punished a large number of times before their self-injurious behavior ceased. They had enough scars on their body. We could not have them continue to mutilate themselves in order that we could treat them! Moreover, the act of carving is usually done in private and is not detected until much later. Accordingly, punishment would have to be delayed, thus lessening its potency. We are not persuaded that punishment can be effective with carving.

It is interesting to attempt to reinterpret aversive conditioning approaches to self-injurious behaviors in terms of co-opting. Speaking metaphorically, when the doctor shocks John for striking himself or banging his head, he may be confusing John as to who is the mutilator–John or the doctor. Who is punishing whom? The doctor seems to be taking over control of John's self-injurious behavior–it is no longer his behavior; no longer a proprietary act; it is behavior which is now controlled by others; John's self-injurious behavior has been co-opted. Similarly it may be that when Lourie (1949) placed a metronome next to a head banging child and set it to match the speed of the child's head banging, the child might have wondered, "Is it me or the metronome that is controlling my behavior?"

In overcorrection procedures (Azrin et al., 1975), in which the autistic child, when observed engaging in self-injurious behavior, is disrupted and required to perform various incompatible behaviors, the patient may feel that his behavior has been, as it were, taken over by his therapist; his behavior is no longer a proprietary act.

We experienced some difficulty in our work with staff who insisted on rewarding the girls for their improved behavior. In spite of our objections, they persisted in offering tangible rewards to our adolescent therapists for their work. Such well-intentioned behavior has no place in co-opting. In co-opting our aim is to encourage our client to behave as an altruistic, concerned helper, with the hope that she will believe she is behaving prosocially not because she is being paid to do so, but because that is the kind of person she is. We wish her to attribute her changed behavior to herself, not to some external agent. Otherwise, when the agent is not present and the concrete rewards are no longer forthcoming, there would be no reason for her to persist in such behavior.

We made the mistake of rewarding some of our adolescent therapists by giving them extra privileges. Each time we did so they quit. They resented being paid off. They saw us as manipulating; themselves as prostituting. "Tipping" them meant we were controlling them.

In training other clinicians to use co-opting, we have found that it is very difficult to counter the very human tendency for the professional to take credit for the success of his clients. The client *must* be able to attribute her changed behavior to her own efforts, not to some external agent.

It is easier to preach co-opting than to practise it.

Before the co-opting program commenced we declared a moratorium on treatment by the psychology staff. No officially sanctioned or formalized treatment programs were introduced as replacements for behavior modification. For several months the professional staff devoted themselves to routine work and to the task of determining what treatment program should be established in the future. Accordingly, during these months we were able to divest ourselves of responsibility for treatment. Were it not for that fact we doubt we could have succeeded in co-opting the girls. We could not have gained control over the girls' behavior if we had continued to be involved in treatment programs which clearly conveyed to them that we were devoted to controlling them. Similarly we could not, while responding to them as therapists, appear to be treating them as patients. We also divested ourselves of all of the administrative duties in the institution which the girls might view as reflecting our attempts to control them. Moreover we disengaged ourselves from the institution's emergency machinery and refused to be drawn into discussions of the girls' psychopathology, antisocial behavior, manipulations, and other topics which were incompatible with the view of the girls we were trying to promote. We would converse only if the topic was related to positive aspects of the girls' behavior and was completely devoid of reference to problems or pathology. As Thumper says in the film *Bambi*, "If you can't say something nice don't say nothing at all."

After the failure of their efforts to engage us in discussions on problems, the staff stopped talking to us. Our behavior created considerable discomfort for us. Our refusal to plan new treatment programs which would be imposed on the girls was interpreted as our being indifferent. We were suspected of doing nothing.

We tried to persuade our professional colleagues and the institutional administrators that the more elaborate treatment programs they were proposing as replacements for the peer oriented approach could augment rather than improve the girls' problems. They would be externally imposed. We persisted in arguing for co-opting as an alternative. This would have entailed a decrease in clinicians' involvement in program matters and a deemphasis on psychodynamically oriented therapy or diagnostic activities. We could only speculate that our ideas were threatening. Perhaps acceptance of our recommendations meant rejecting traditional roles, accepting reduced authority and responsibility, and living with lessened status. Implied by our comments was the conclusion that clinicians were not needed; their patients could get along with them. Co-opting was preempted.

There followed a resurgence of old programs such as individual and group psychotherapy, behavior modification, and the introduction of some new programs. There also followed a resurgence of carving.

We should have co-opted our colleagues.

Epilogue

Grandview Training School was officially closed on July 6, 1976.

References

Alderson, M.R. Self-poisoning - what is the future? *Lancet*, May 25, 1974, pp. 1040-1043.

Allen, K.E., and Harris, F.R. Elimination of a child's excessive scratching by training the mother in reinforcement procedures. *Behaviour Research and Therapy*, 1966, 4:79-84.

Asch, S.S. Wrist scratching as a symptom of anhedonia; a pre-depressive state. *Psychoanalytic Quarterly*, 1971, 40:603-613.

Atkins, R.A. *Personal communication*, 1978.

Azrin, N.H., Gottlieb, I., Hughart, L., Wesolowski, M.D., and Rahn, T. Eliminating self-injurious behaviour by educative procedures. *Behaviour Research and Therapy*, 1975, 13(2-3):101-111.

Bachman, J.A. Self-injurious behaviour—a behavioural analysis. *Journal of Abnormal Psychology*, 1972, 80(3):211-224.

Bach-Y-Rita, G. Habitual violence and self-mutilation. *American Journal of Psychiatry*, 1974, 131(9):1018-1020.

Bach-Y-Rita, G., and Veno A. Habitual violence: A profile of 62 men. *American Journal of Psychiatry*, 1974, 131(9):1015-1017.

Bagley, C. Authoritarianism, status integration, and suicide. *Sociology*, 1972, 6(3):395-404.

Bagley, C. Social policy and the prevention of suicidal behaviour. *British Journal of Social Work*, 1973 3(4):473-495.

Bagley, C. and Greer, S. Clinical and social predictors of repeated attempted suicide; A multivariate analysis. *British Journal of Psychiatry*, 1971, 119:515-521.

Bagley, C., and Greer, S. "Black suicide": A report of 25 English cases and controls. *Journal of Social Psychology*, 1972, 86:175-179.

Bagley, C., Jacobson, S., and Rehin, A. Completed suicide: a taxonomic analysis of clinical and social data. *Psychological Medicine*, 1976, 6:429-438.

Ball, T.S. Issues and implications of operant conditioning: the reestablishment of social behavior. *Hospital and Community Behavior*, 1968,19:230-232.

Ball, T.S., Sibback, L., Jones, R., Steele, B., and Frazier, L. An accelerometer-activated device to control assaultive and self-destructive behaviours in retardates. *Journal of Behaviour Therapy and Experimental Psychiatry*, 1975, 6(3):223-228.

Ballinger, B.R. The prevalence of nail-biting in normal and abnormal populations. *British Journal of Psychiatry*, 1970, 117:445-446.

Ballinger, B.R. Minor self-injury. *British Journal of Psychiatry*, 1971, 118:535-538.

Bancroft, J.H., Skrimshire, A.N., Reynolds, F., Simkin, S., and Smith, J. Self-poisoning and self-injury in the Oxford area: Epidemiological aspects 1969-1973. *British Journal of Preventive and Social Medicine*, 1975, 29(3):170-177.

Bandura, A. *Principles of Behavior Modification.* New York:Holt, Rinehart and Winston, 1969.

Baroff, G.S. On the use of aversive techniques in controlling self-injurious behavior. *American Psychologist*. 1976, p. 616.

Battle, R.J.V. and Marshall, H.E.S. Attempted suicide by burning. *British Medical Journal*, Dec. 27, 1952, pp. 1397-1398.

Battle, R.J.V., and Pollitt, J.D. Self-inflicted injuries. *British Journal of Plastic Surgery*, 1964, 17:400-412.

Bean, P. Patterns of self-poisoning. *British Journal of Preventive and Social Medicine*, 1974, 28:24-31.

Bem, D. Self-perception: An alternative interpretation of cognitive dissonance phenomena. *Psychological Review*, 1967, 74:183-200.

Bergman, R.L. Behavioral contracting with chronic schizophrenics. *Journal of Behaviour Therapy and Experimental Psychiatry*, 1975, 6:355-356.

Berkow, R. Difficult definition of malingering. *New England Journal of Medicine*, 1970, 283:710.

Berkson,G., and Davenport, R.K. Stereotyped movements of mental defectives. *American Journal of Mental Deficiency*, 1964, 68:511-524.

Bettelheim, B. *Symbolic Wounds*. Glencoe: Free Press, 1954.

Betts, W.C. Autocannibalism. *American Journal of Psychiatry*, 1964, 121:402-403.

Blacker, K.H., and Wong, N. Four cases of autocastration. *Archives of General Psychiatry*, 1963, 8:169-174.

Bostic, R.A. Self-immolation: A survey of the last decade. *Life Threateing Behavior,* 1973, 3(1):66-74.

Bowlby, J. *Maternal Care and Mental Health*. Geneva: World Health Organization, 1952.

Brawley, E.R., Harris, F.R., Allen, K.E., Fleming, R.S., and Peterson, R.F. Behavior modification of an autistic child. *Behavioral Science*, 1969, 14:87-97.

Brenman, M. On teasing and being teased: and the problem of moral masochism. *Psychoanalytic Study of the Child*, 1952, 7:264-285.

Brown, J.S., Martin, R. C., and Morrow, M.W. Self-punitive behavior in the rat: facilitative effects of punishment on resistance to extinction. *Journal of Comparative and Physiological Psychology*, 1964, 57(1):127-133.

Bryson, Y., Sakati, N., Nyhan, W.L., and Fish, C.H. Self-mutilative behaviour in the Cornelia de Lange syndrome. *American Journal of Mental Deficiency*, 1971, 76(3):319-324.

Bucher, B., and Lovaas, O.I. Use of aversive stimulation in behavior modification. In M. Jones (Ed.) *Miami Symposium on the prediction of behavior.* 1967:Coral Gables, Fla.:University of Miami Press, 1968.

Buglass, D., and Horton, J. A scale for predicting subsequent suicidal behavior. *British Journal of Psychiatry*, 1974 124:573-578.

Burchard, J.D., and Tyler, V. The modification of delinquent behavior through operant conditioning. *Behavior Research and Therapy*, 1965, 2:245-250.

Burnham, R.C. Symposium on impulsive self-mutilation: Discussion. *British Journal of Medical Psychology*, 1969, 42:233.

Carr, E.G. The motivation of self-injurious behavior: A review of some hypotheses. *Psychological Bulletin*, 1977, 84:800-816.

Carson, D., and Lewis, J.M. Ocular auto-enucleation while under the influence of drugs: A case report. *Adolescence*, 1971, 6(23):397-403.

Carson, R.C. *An Introduction to M.M.P.I. Interpretation*. Duke University, 1960.

Cautela, J, and Baron, M. Multifacetted behaviour therapy of self-injurious behaviour. *Journal of Behaviour Therapy and Experimental Psychiatry*, 1973, 4:125-131.

Claghorn, J.L., and Beto, S.R. Self-mutilation in a prison hospital. *Corrective Psychiatry and Journal of Social Therapy*, 1967, 13:133-140.

Clanon, T.L. Persecutory feelings and self-mutilation in prisoners. *Corrective Psychiatry and Journal of Social Therapy*, 1965, 11:96-102.

Cohen, H.L., and Philipczak, *J. A New Learning Environment*. San Francisco: Jossey-Bass, 1971.

Collins, D.T. Head banging: its meaning and management in the severely retarded adult. *Bulletin of the Menninger Clinic*, 1965, 4:205-211.

Cookson, H.M. A survey of self-injury in a closed prison for women. *British Journal of Ciminology,* 1977, 17(4):332-357.

Cooper, A.F., and Fowlie, H.C. Control of gross self-mutilation by lithium carbonate. *British Journal of Psychiatry*, 1973, 122:370.

Cohen, R.J. Comments on the "cattle-prod controversy." *Perceptual and Motor Skills*, 1976, 42:146.

Cormack, G. Personal communication, 1968.

Corte, H.E., Wolff, M.M. and Locke, B.J. Comparison of procedures for eliminating self-injurious behaviour of retarded adolescents. *Journal of Applied Behaviour Analysis*, 1971, (4):201-207.

Cox, M., and Klinge, V. Treatment and management of a case of self-burning. *Behaviour Research and Therapy,* 1976, 14(5):382-385.

Crabtree, L., Jr. A psycho-therapeutic encounter with a self-mutilating patient. *Psychiatry*, 1967, 30:91-100.

Crabtree, L., Jr., and Grossman, W. Administrative clarity and redefinition for an open adolescent unit. *Psychiatry*, 1974, 37:350-359.

Critchley, M. Some aspects of pain. *British Medical Journal*, 1934, 2:891.

Critchley, M. Congenital indifference to pain. *Annals of Internal Medicine*, 1956, 45:737-747.

Davidson, S.I. Auto-enucleation of the eye: A study of self-mutilation. *Acta Psychotherapy*, 1962, 10:286-300.

de Lange, C. Sur un type nouveau de degeneration (Typus amstelodamensis). *Archives Medicin des Enfants*, 1933, 36:713.

DeLissovoy, V. Head banging in early childhood: A study of incidence. *Journal of Pediatrics,* 1961, 58:803-805.

DeLissovoy, V. Head banging in early childhood. *Child Development*, 1962, 33:43-56.

Duker, P. Behaviour control of self-biting in a Lesch-Nyhan patient. *Journal of Mental Deficiency Research*, 1975, 19(1):11-19.

Dunlap, K. *Habits: Their Making and Unmaking*. New York: Liveright, 1932.

Edmonson, J.S. A case of sexual asphyxia without fatal termination. *British Journal of Psychiatry*, 1972, 121:437-438.

Egan, G. *The Skilled Helper*. Monterey, Calif.: Brooks/Cole, 1975.

Ernst, F.A. Self-recording and counterconditioning of a self-mutilative compulsion. *Behavior Therapy*, 1973, 4:144-146.

Evans, J.G. Deliberate self-poisoning in the Oxford area. *British Journal of Preventive Medicine*, 1967, 21:97-107.

Fenichel, O. *The Psychoanalytical Theory of Neurosis*. New York: Norton, 1945.

Ferenczi, S. The unwelcome child and his death instinct. In *Final Contributions to the Problems and Methods and Psychoanalysis*. New York: Basic Books, 1956.

Ferrence, R.G., and Johnson, F.G. Factors affecting reported rates of self-injury. *Life-Threatening Behavior*, 1974, 4(1):54-66.

Ferster, C.B. *Behavior Principles*. New York: Appleton-Century-Crofts, 1968.

Fielding, L.T., and Cole, S.M. Recording observations of self-injurious behaviour. *Mental Retardation*, 1971, 9(3):31.

Foster, T.M. Make-believe families: a response of women and girls to the deprivation of imprisonment. *International Journal of Criminology and Penology,* 1975, 3:71-78.

Foxx, R.M., and Azrin, N.H. The elimination of autistic self-stimulatory behaviour by overcorrection. *Journal of Applied Behavior Analysis*, 1973, 6:1-14.

Frankel, B., Ferrence, R., Johnson, F., and Whitehead, P. Drinking and self-injury: Toward untangling the dynamics. *British Journal of Addiction,* 1976, 71:299-306.

Frankl, V.E. Paradoxical intention: a logotherapeutic technique. *American Journal of Psychotherapy*, 1960, 14:520-535.

Frankel, F., and Simmons, J.Q. Self-injurious behavior in schizophrenic and retarded children. *American Journal of Mental Deficiency*, 1976, 80:512-522.

French, A.P., and Nelson, H.L. Genital self-mutilation in women. *Archives of General Psychiatry*, 1972, 27:618-620.

Freidman, M., Glasser, M. Laufer, E., Laufer, M., and Wohl, M. Attempted suicide and self-mutilation in adolescents: Some observations from a psychoanalytic research project. *International Journal of Psychological Analysis*, 1972, 53(2):179-183.

Gardner, J.E. Behaviour therapy treatment approach to a psychogenic seizure case. *Journal of Consulting Psychology*, 1965, 31:209-212.

Gardner, A.R., and Gardner, A.J. Self-mutilation, obsessionality, and narcissim. *British Journal of Psychiatry*, 1975, 127:127-132.

Gendreau, P., and Ross, R.R. Effective correctional treatment: bibliotherapy for cynics. *Crime and Delinquency*, 1979 (in press)

Gesell, A., and Ilg, F.L. Infant and child in the culture of today. *Harper*, 1943.

Gioviacchini, P.L. Defensive meaning of a specific anxiety syndrome. *Psychoanalytic Review,* 1956, 43:373-380.

Glasser, W. *Reality Therapy: A new Approach to Psychiatry.* New York: Harper and Row, 1965.

Gold, S.R., and Coghlan, A.J. Locus of control and self-esteem among adolescent drug abusers: effects of residential treatment. *Drug Forum*, 1975-76, 5(2):185-191.

Goldfarb, W. Pain reactions in a group of institutionalized schizophrenic children. *American Journal of Orthopsychiatry,* 1958, 28:775-785.

Goldfield, M., and Glick, I. Self-mutilation of the female genitalia. *Diseases of the Nervous System,* 1970, 31(12):843-845.

Goldney, R.D., and Simpson, I.G. Female genital self-mutilation, dysorexia and the hysterical personality: The Caenis syndrome. *Journal of the Canadian Psychiatric Association*, 1975, 20:435-441.

Goodhart, S.P., and Savitsky, N. Self-mutilation in chronic encephalitis. *American Journal Medical Science,* 1933, 185:674.

Graff, H., and Mallin, R. The syndrome of the wrist cutter. *American Journal of Psychiatry*, 1967, 124:36-42.

Green, A.H. Self-mutilation in schizophrenic children. *Archives of General Psychiatry*, 1967, 17:234-244.

Green, A.H. Self-destructive behaviour in physically abused, schizophrenic children. *Archives of General Psychiatry,* 1968, 19:171-178.

Greer, S., and Lee, H.A. Subsequent progress of potentially lethal attempted suicides. *Acta Psychiatrica Scandinavica*, 1967, 43:361-371.

Guerney, B.G. Psychotherapeutic *Agents: New Roles for Nonprofessionals, Parents, And Teacher*. New York: Holt, Rinehart and Winston, 1969.

Haley, J. *Uncommon Therapy: The Psychiatric Techniques of Milton H. Erikson, M.D.* New York: Norton, 1973.

Hamilton, J., Stephens, L. and Allen, P. Controlling aggressive and destructive behavior in severely retarded institutionalized residents. *American Journal of Mental Deficiency*, 1967, 71:852-856.

Harlow, H.F. Early social deprivation and later behavior in the monkey. In A. Abrams, H. Garner, and J. Toman (eds), *Unfinished Tasks in the Behavioral Sciences*. Baltimore: Williams and Wilkins, 1964.

Harlow, H.F., and Suomi, S.J. Induced psychopathology in monkeys. *Engineering and Science*, 1970, 33:8-14.

Harris, C.N., and Raik, K. Self-inflicted wrist slash. *Journal of Trauma*, 1976, 16(9):743-745.

Hartman, H. Self-mutilation. *Janrb. F. Psychiat. u. Neurol.*, 1925, 44:31: Abstracted by Keschner, *Archives of Neurology and Psychiatry*, 1926, 15:384-386.

Hatton, C.L., Valenti, S.M., and Rink, A. *Suicide: Assessment and Intervention.* New York: Appleton-Century-Crofts, 1977.

Hawkins, J.R., Jones, K., and Tibbetts, R.W. Deliberate disability. *British Medical Journal,* 1956, 1:(361).

Helzel, M. Personal communication, 1978.

Hinsie, L.E., and Campbell, R.J. *Psychiatric Dictionary.* New York: Oxford University Press, 1960.

Hoefnagel, D.A., Donald, F., Mireault, N.G. and Berndt, W.O. Hereditary choreoathetosis, self-mutilation and hyperuricemia in young males. *New England Journal of Medicine*, 1965, 273:13-135.

Holz, W.D., and Azrin, N.K. Discriminative properties of punishment. *Journal of Experimental Analysis of Behaviour*, 1961, 4:225-232.

The Interpreters' Dictionary of the Bible, vol. 1-4, Nashville, Tenn.: Abingdon Press, 1962.

Jacobson, S., and Tribe, P. Deliberate self-injury (attempted suicide) in patients admitted to hospital in mid-Sussex. *British Journal of Psychiatry*, 1972, 121: 379.

Jarvis, G., Ferrence, R., Johnson, G., and Whitehead, P. Sex and patterns in self-injury. *Journal of Health and Social Behavior*, 1976, 17(2):145-155.

Jayewardene, C.H.S. Personal communication, 1978.

Johnson, E.H. Felon self-mutilation: Correlates of stress in prison. In B.L. Danto (ed.), *Jailhouse Blues.* Orchard Lake, Mich.: Epic Publications, 1973.

Johnson, G., Ferrence, R. and Whitehead, P. Self-injury: identification and intervention. *Canadian Psychiatric Association Journal*, 1973, 18:101-105.

Johnson, F.G., Frankel, B.G., Ferrence, R.G., Jarvis, G.K., and Whitehead, P.C. Self-injury in London, Canada: A prospective study. *Canadian Journal of Public Health*, 1975, 66:307-316.

Johnson, W. *People in Quandries: The Semantics of Personal Adjustment*. New York: Harper and Row, 1946.

Jones, D.A. *The Health Risks of Imprisonment.* Lexington, Mass.: D.C. Heath, 1976.

Jones, F.H., Simmons, J., and Frankel, F. An extinction procedure for elimi-nationg self-destructive behaviour in a 9-year old autistic girl. *Journal of Autism and Childhood Schizophrenia,* 1974, 4(3):241-250.

Kafka, J.S. The body as transitional object: a psychoanalytic study of a self-mutilating patient. *British Journal of Medical Psychology,* 1969, 42:207-212.

Kafka, J.S. Ambiguity for individuation: A critique and reformation of double-bind theory. *Archives of General Psychiatry,* 1971, 25:223-239.

Kessel, N. The respectability of self-poisoning and the fashion of survival. *Journal of Psychosomatic Research,* 1966, 10:29-36.

Korten, J.J., Van Dorp, A., Hustinx, T.W., Scheres, J.M., and Rutten, F. J. Self-mutilation in a case of 49,XXXY chromosonal constitution. *Journal of Mental Deficiency Research,* March 1975, 63-71.

Kravitz, H., Rosenthal, V., Teplitz, Z., Murphy, J.B., and Lesser, R.E. A study of head banging in infants and children. *Disease of the Nervous System,* 1960, 21:203-208.

Laing, R.D., and Esternson, A. *Sanity, Madness and the Family.* London: Tavistock, 1964.

Lazarus, A. *Behavior Therapy and Beyond.* New York: McGraw-Hill, 1971.

Lefcourt, H.M. *Locus of Control: Current Trends in Theory and Research.* New York: Halstead Press, 1976.

Lesch, M., and Nyhan, W.L. A familiar disorder of uric acid metabolism and central nervous system function. *American Journal of Medicine,* 1964, 36:561.

Lester, D. Self-mutilating behavior. *Psychological Bulletin,* 1972, 78(2):119-128.

Lester, G., and Lester, D. *Suicide: The Gamble with Death.* Englewood Cliffs, N.J.: Prentice-Hall, 1971.

Levy, D.M. On the problem of movement restraint. *American Journal of Orthopsychiatry,* 1944, 14:644-671.

Levy, D.M., and Patrick, H.T. Relation of infantile convulsions, head banging and breath holding to fainting and headaches in the parents. *Archives of Neurology and Psychiatry,* 1949, 105: 653-660.

Levy, L.H. *Psychological Interpretation.* New York: Holt, Rinehart and Winston, 1963.

Lourie, R.S. The role of rhythmic patterns in childhood. *American Journal of Psychiatry,* 1949, 105:653-660.

Lovaas, O.I., Freitag, G., Gold, V., and Kassorla, I. Experimental studies in childhood schizophrenia: Analysis of self-destructive behaviour. *Journal of Experimental Child Psychology,* 1965, 2:67-84.

Lovaas, O.I., Schaeffer, B., and Simmons, J. Experimental studies in childhood schizophrenia: building social behavior in autistic children by the use of electric shock. *Journal of Experimental Research in Personality,* 1965, 1:99-109.

Lovaas, O.I., and Simmons, J. Manipulation of self-destruction in three retarded children. *Journal of Applied Behaviour Analysis,* 1969, 2:143-157.

Lubin, A.J. Vincent van Gogh's ear. *Psychoanalytic Quarterly,* 1961, 30:351-384.

Lucero, W.J., Frieman, J., Spoering, K., and Fehrenbacher, J. Comparison of three procedures in reducing self-injurious behavior. *American Journal of Mental Deficiency,* 1976, 180(5):548-554.

MacGuigan, Mark (chairman). *Report on the Sub-Committee on Penitentiaries in Canada.* Ottawa: Ministry of Supply and Services, 1977.

McKerracher, D., Loughane, T., and Watson, R. Self-mutilation in female psychopaths. *British Journal of Psychiatry,* 1968, 14:829-832.

McNeil, G., and Vance, S. *Cruel and Unusual.* Toronto: Deneau and Greenberg Publishers, 1978.

Marks, I.M., Rachman, S., and Gelder, M.G. Methods for assessment of aversion treatment in fetishism with masochism. *Behavioral Research and Therapy,* 1965, 3:253-258.

Martin, G., and Treffry, D. Treating self-destruction and developing self-care with a severely retarded girl: A case study. *Psychological Aspects of Disability,* 1970, 17(3):125-131.

Matthews, P.C. Epidemic self-injury in an adolescent unit. *International Journal of Social Psychiatry,* 1968, 14:125-133.

Menninger, K. A psychoanalytic study of the significance of self-mutilations. *Psychoanalytic Quarterly,* 1935, 4:408-466.

Menninger, K.A. *Man against Himself.* New York: Harcourt Brace, 1938.

Merbaum, M. Modification of self-destructive behaviour by a mother therapist using aversive stimuli. *Behaviour Therapy,* 1973, 4:442-447.

Michael, K.D., and Beck, R. Self-amputation of the tongue. *International Journal of Psychoanalytic Psychotherapy,* 1973, 2(1):93-99.

Miller, F., and Bashkin, E. Depersonalization and self-mutilation. *Psychoanalytic Quarterly,* 1974, 43(4):638-649.

Mintz, I.L. Autocannibalism. *American Journal of Psychiatry,* 1964, 120:1017.

Mishara, B.L., Robertson, B., and Kastenbaum, R. Self-injurious behavior in the elderly. *Gerontologist,* 1973, 1:311-314.

Mitchell, G. What monkeys can tell us about human violence. *Futurist,* April 1975, 75-80.

Money, J., Wolff, G., and Annecillo, C. Pain agnosia and self-injury in the syndrome of reversible somatotropin deficiency (psychosocial dwarfism). *Journal of Autism and Childhood Schizophrenia,* 1972, 2(2):127-139.

Morgan, H.G., Burns-Cox, C.H., Pocock, H., and Pottle, S. Deliberate self-harm: clinical and socio-economic characteristics of 368 patients. *British Journal of Psychiatry,* 1975 127:564-574.

Morgan, H.G., Pocock, H., and Pottle, S. The urban distribution of non-fatal deliberate self-harm. *British Journal of Psychiatry,* 1975, 126:319-328.

Morgan, H.G., Barton, J., and Pottle, S. Deliberate self-harm: A follow-up study of 179 patients. *British Journal of Psychiatry,* 1976, 128:361-368.

Morrison, D. Issues in the application of reinforcement theory in the treatment of a child's self-injurious behaviour. *Psychotherapy: Theory, Research and Practice,* 1972, 9(1):40-45.

Murray, M. and Nevin, J.A. Shock effects of correlation between response-contingent shock and reinforcement. *Journal of the Experimetnal Analysis of Behavior,* 1967, 10:301-309.

Muttar, A., Peck, A., Whitlow, D., and Fraser, W. Reversal of a severe case of self-mutilation. *Journal of Mental Deficiency Research,* 1975, 19(3):3-9.

Myers, D.V. Case histories and shorter communications. *Behaviour Research and Therapy,* 1975, 13:189-191.

Myers, J.J., and Deibert, A. Reduction of self-abusive behaviour in a blind child by using a feeding response. *Journal of Behaviour Therapy and Experimental Psychiatry,* 1971, 2:141-144.

National Institute of Education. *Violent Schools–Safe Schools,* vol. 1. Washington D.C.: U.S. Department of Health, Education and Welfare, 1978.

Neil, J.F. Self-mutilation of the tongue. *Journal of Larynology,* 1958, 72:947-950.

Neill, A.S. *Summerhill: A Radical Approach to Child Rearing.* New York:Hart, 1960.

Nelson, S., and Grunebaum, H. A follow-up study of wrist slashers. *American Journal of Psychiatry,* 1971, 127:1345-1349.

New Catholic Encyclopedia, vols. 1-15. New York: McGraw-Hill, 1967.

Novotny, P. Self-cutting. *Bulletin of the Menninger Clinic,* 1972, 36(5):505-514.

Nyhan, W.L., and Lesch, M. A familiar disorder of uric acid metabolism and central nervous system function. *American Journal of Medicine,* 1964, 36:561.

Offer, D., and Barlow, P. Adolescent and young adult self-mutilation incidents in a general psychiatric hospital. *Archives of General Psychiatry,* 1960, 3:194-204.

Olsen, J. Self-inflicted injuries and false information to the police. *Medicine, Science and the Law,* 1967, 7:22-25.

Panton, J. The identification of predispositional factors in self-mutilation within a state prison population. *Journal of Clinical Psychology,* 1962, 18:63-67.

Pao, P. The syndrome of delicate self-cutting. *British Journal of Medical Psychology,* 1969, 42:195-205.

Parker, C.E., Mavalwala, J., Weise, P., Koch, R., Hatashita, A., and Cibilich, S. The 47,XYY syndrome in a boy with behavior problems and mental retardation. *American Journal of Mental Deficiency,* 1970, 74:660.

Peterson, R., and Peterson, L. The use of positive reinforcement in the control of self-destructive behaviour in a retarded boy. *Journal of Experimental Child Psychology,* 1968, 3:351-360.

Phillips, R., and Alkan, M. Some aspects of self-mutilation in the general population of a large psychiatric hospital. *Psychological Quarterly,* 1961, 35:421-423.

Phillips, R.H., and Muzaffer, A. Some aspects of self-mutilation in the general population of a large psychiatric hospital. *Psychiatric Quarterly,* 1961, 35:421-423.

Pindborg, J.J., Dental mutilation and associated abnormalities in Uganda. *American Journal of Physical Anthropology,* 1969, 31:383-390.

Podvoll, E.M. Self-mutilation within a hospital setting: A study of identity and social compliance. *British Journal of Medical Psychology,* 1969, 42:213-221.

Rado, S. Fear of castration in women. *Psychoanalytic Quarterly,* 1933, 2:425-75.

Ragain, R.D., and Anson, J.E. The control of self-mutilating behavior with positive reinforcement. *Mental Retardation,* 1976, 14(3):22-25.

Rechter, E., and Vrablic, M. The right to treatment including aversive stimuli. *Psychiatric Quarterly,* 1974, 48 (3):445-449.

Repp, A.C., and Deitz, S.M. Reducing aggressive and self-injurious behavior of institutionalized retarded children through reinforcement of other behavior. *Journal of Applied Behavior Analysis,* 1974, 7:313-325.

Ressman, A.C., and Butterworth, T. Localized acquired hypertrichosis. *Archives of Dermatology and Syphillis,* 1952, 65:458-423.

Riessman, F. The Helper Therapy Principle. *Social Work,* 1965, 10:27-65.

Risley, T.R. The effects and side effects of punishing the autistic behaviors of a deviant child. *Journal of Applied Behavior Analysis,* 1968, (1):21-34.

Roback, H., Frayn, D., Gunby, L., and Tuters, K. A multifactorial approach to the treatment and ward management of a self-mutilating patient. *Journal of Behaviour Therapy and Experimental Psychiatry,* 1972, 3(3):189-193.

Romanczyk, R.G., and Goren, E. Severe self-injurious behaviour: The problem of clinical control. *Journal of Consulting and Clinical Psychology,* 1975, 43(5):730-739.

Rosenthal, R., and Jacobson, L. *Pygmalion in the Classroom.* New York: Holt, Rinehart and Winston, 1968.

Rosenthal, R.J., Rinzler, C., Walsh, R., and Klausner, E. Wrist cutting syndrome: the meaning of a gesture. *American Journal of Psychiatry,* . 1972, 128(11):47-52.

Ross, R.R., *Behavioral Management in the Control and Treatment of the Offender.* Ottawa: University of Ottawa Press, 1977.

Ross, R.R., *Rewards for offenders.* Paper presented at Symposium on New Trends in Criminology, Simon Fraser University, Vancouver, B.C., April 1975.

Ross, R.R., Meichenbaum, D.H., and Humphreys, C. Treatment of nocturnal head banging by behavior modification techniques. *Behavior Research and Therapy,* 1971, 9:151-154.

Ross, R.R., and Doody, K. Persistence in the psychopathic personality. *Canadian Journal of Criminology and Corrections,* 1973, 15:292-305.

Ross, R.R., and McKay, H.B. Behavior modification and the offender therapist: Are they compatible? Paper presented at Annual Meeting of Canadian Psychological Association, Quebec City, 1975.

Ross, R.R., and McKay, H.B. A study of institutional treatment programs. *International Journal of Offender Therapy and Comparative Criminology,* 176(a), 20:165-173.

Ross, R.R., and McKay, H.B. Adolescent therapists. *Canada's Mental Health,* 1976(b), 24(2):15-17.

Ross, R.R., and Price, M.J. Behavior modification in corrections: Autopsy before mortification. *International Journal of Criminology and Penology,* 1976, 4:305-315.

Ross, R.R., and McKay, H.B. Behavioral approaches to treatment in corrections: Requiem for a panacea. *Canadian Journal of Criminology,* 1978(a) 20:279-295.

Ross, R.R., and McKay, H.B. Positive and negative operant conditioning with female adolescent offenders. *Acta Criminologica Japanica et Medicinae Legale,* 1978(b) 44:54-64.

Ryback, R.S. Self-mutilation during alcoholic amnesia–report of a case. *British Journal of Psychiatry,* 1971, 118-(546):535.

Sandler, J. Masochism: An empirical analysis. *Psychological Bulletin,* 1964, 62(2):197-204.

Sandow, S. Study of informal approaches to treatment of self-injurious behaviour in the severely subnormal. *British Journal of Mental Subnormality,* 1975, 21(40):10-17.

Saposnek, D., and Watson, L. The elimination of the self-destructive behaviour of a psychotic child: a case study. *Behaviour Therapy,* 1974, 5:79-89.

Schaefer, H.H. Self-injurious behavior: Shaping "head banging" in monkeys. *Journal of Applied Behavior Analysis,* 1970, 3:111-116.

Schott, G. Selbstkastration aus sadisticher triebpecrecsion, zugleich ein Beitrag zur Antiandiogentherapie. *Psychiat. Neurol. Med. Psychol.,* 1973, 25:435-442.

Schwitzgebel, R.L. Preliminary socialization for psychotherapy of behavior-disordered adolescents. *Journal of Consulting and Clinical Psychology,* 1969, 33:71-77.

Scott, G.D. The prisoner of society: Psychiatric syndromes in captive society. *Correctional Psychologist,* 1969, 3:3-5.

Sears, R., Moccoby, E., and Levin, H. *Patterns of Child Rearing.* New York: Harper and Row, 1957.

Segal, P., Mrzyglod, S., Alichniewicz-Cz plicka, H., Dunin-Horokawicz, W., and Zwyrzykowski, E. Self-inflicted eye injuries. *American Journal of Opthalomology,* 1963, 55:349-362.

Shah, D.K., and Rohter, W. Brazil's bizarre cults. *Newsweek,* February 27, 1978, p. 86.

Shaver, K.G. *An Introduction to Attribution Processes.* Cambridge, Mass.: Winthrop Publishers, 1975.

Shear, C.S., Nyhan, W., Kirman, B.H., and Stern, J. Self-mutilative behavior as a feature of the de Lange Syndrome. *Journal of Pediatrics,* 1971, 78:506-509.

Shintoub, S.A., and Soulairac, A. L'enfant auto-mutilateur. *Psychiatrie Enfant,* 1961, 3:119.

Shodell, M.J., and Reiter, H.H. Self-mutilative behaviour in verbal and nonverbal schizophrenic children. *Archives of General Psychiatry,* 1968, 19:453-455.

Simpson, M. Female genital self-mutilation. *Archives of General Psychiatry,* 1973, 29:808-810.

Simpson, M.A. The phenomenology of self-mutilation in a general hospital setting. *Canadian Psychiatric Association Journal,* 1975, 20(6):429-433.

Singh, N.N. Psychological treatment of self-injury. *New Zealand Medical Journal,* 1976, 84(578):484-486.

Siomopoulos, V. Repeated self-cutting: An impulse neurosis. *American Journal of Psychotherapy,* 1974, 28:85-94.

Sjoberg, L. Alcohol and gambling. *Psychopharmacologia,* 1969, 14:284-298.

Skinner, B.F. *Science and Human Behavior.* New York: Macmillan, 1953.

Skrimshire, A.M. A small area analysis of self-poisoning and self-injury in the region of Oxford. *Journal of Biosocial Science,* 1976, 8:85-112.

Slawson, P., and Davidson, P. Hysterical self-mutilation of the tongue. *Archives of General Psychiatry,* 1964, 11:581-588.

Smolev, S. Use of operant techniques for the modification of self-injurious behavior. *American Journal of Mental Deficiency,* 1971, 76:295-305.

Spitz, R. Hospitalism. *Psychoanalytic Study of the Child,* 1945, 1:53-74.

Spitz, R.A., and Wolf, K.M. Anaclitic depression. *Psychoanalytic Study of the Child,* 1946, 2:313-342.

Steffy, R.A., Hart, J., and Craw, M. Behavior modification treatment with young adult aggressive patients: A case report. Paper presented at Ontario Psychological Association, February 1967.

Stekel, W. *Auto-erotism: A Psychiatric Study of Onanism and Neurosis.* New York: Grove Press, 1961.

Stengel, E., and Cook, N.C. *Attempted Suicide: Its Social Significance and Effects.* London: Chapman and Hall, 1958.

Stinnett, J.L. and Hollender, M.H. Compulsive self-mutilation. *Journal of Nervous and Mental Diseases,* 1970, 150(5):371.

Stuart, R.B. *Trick or Treatment: How and When Psychotherapy Fails.* Champaign, Ill. Research Press, 1970.

Szasz, T. The Myth of Mental Illness. New York: Harper and Row, 1961.

Tanner, B.A., and Zeiler, M. Punishment of self injurious behavior using aromatic amonia as the averse stimulus. *Journal of Applied Behavior Analysis,* 1975, 8(1).

Tate, B.G. Case study: Control of chronic self-injurious behaviour by conditioning procedure. *Behaviour Therapy,* 1972 3(1):72-83.

Tate, B.G., and Baroff, G.S. Aversive control of self-injurious behavior in a psychotic boy. *Behavior Research and Therapy,* 1966, 4:281-287.

Taylor, A.J.W. The significance of "darls" as special relationships for borstal girls. *British Journal of Criminology,* 1965, 5:406-418.

Tyler, V.O. Application of operant token reinforcement to academic performance of an institutionalized delinquent. *Psychological Reports,* 1967, 21:249-260.

Varga, E., and Simpson, G.M. Loxapine succinate in the treatment of uncontrollable destructive behavior. *Current Therapeutic Research,* 1971, 13(12):737-741.

Virkkunen, M. Self-mutilation in antisocial personality (disorder). *Acta Psychiatrica Scandinavica,* 1976, 54:347-352.

Wechsler, D. The incidence and significance of finger-nail biting in children. *Psychoanalytic Review,* 1931, 18:201-209.

Weiher, R.G., and Harman, R.E. The use of omission training to reduce self-injurious behavior in a retarded child. *Behavior Therapy,* 1975, 6:261-268.

Whitehead, P., and Ferrence, R. Measuring the incidence of self-injury: some methodological and design considerations. *American Journal of Orthopsychiatry,* 1973(a), 43(1):142-148.

Whitehead, P., and Ferrence, R. Physicians' reports of self-injury cases among their patients not seen in the hospital. *Life-Threatening Behaviour,* 1973(b), 3(2):137-146.

Whitehead, P.C., Johnson, F.G., Ferrence, R. Measuring the incidence of self-inury: some methodological and design considerations. *American Journal of Orthopsychiatry,* 1973, 43:(1).

Wilbur, R.L., Chandler, P.J., and Carpenter, B.L. Modification of self-injurious behavior by aversive conditioning. *Behavioral Engineering,* 1974, 1:14-25.

Williams, C.E. Self-injury in children. Developmental Medicine and Child Neurology, 1974, 16:88-90.

Wolff, M.M., Risley, T., and Mees, H. Application of operant conditioning procedures to the behavior problems of an autistic child. *Behavior Research and Therapy,* 1964, 1:305-312.

Wright, L. Aversive conditioning of self-induced seizures. *Behavior Therapy,* 1973, 4:712-713.

Yaroshevsky, F. Self-mutilation in soviet prisons. *Canadian Psychiatric Association Journal,* 1975, 20(6):443-446.

Zimbardo, P.G. A social-psychological analysis of vandalism: Making sense of senseless violence. *ONR Tehcnical Report,* Z-05, Dec. 1970.

Author Index

Subject Index

About the Authors

Robert Robertson Ross is professor of criminology, University of Ottawa. He received the Ph.D. in psychology from the University of Toronto. Dr. Ross has been research associate, human justice program, University of Regina; lecturer, Wilfred Laurier University; and associate professor of psychology, University of Waterloo. His experience in criminal justice is extensive and includes more than ten years as clinical psychologist in a wide variety of correctional institutions for juveniles and adults. For twelve years he was chief psychologist for the Ontario Government's Ministry of Correctional Services. He has also been a faculty member for the Ontario Department of Education's programs for special education teachers, and a consultant to the Department of Educational Television. He is the recipient of the Atkinson Foundation Fellowship and the Centennial Medal of Canada. Dr. Ross's publications include numerous articles in professional journals in psychology, criminology, and corrections, and chapters in several books on behavior modification and corrections.

Hugh Bryan McKay is assistant professor of criminology in the Faculty of Social Sciences at the University of Ottawa. As a Canada Council Doctoral Fellow he received his graduate training in clinical and social psychology at the University of Waterloo. His professional experience in the criminal justice field is extensive, spanning more than a decade of research, teaching, and practice. Currently an associate editor of the journal *Crime et/and Justice*, he also serves as a consultant on criminal justice matters to federal and provincial government agencies, advisory groups, and professional associations in the law enforcement and corrections field. His most recent publications include work on prison riots, the effects of long-term imprisonment, theories of social justice, and criminal justice policy and management issues.